LIFE BEGINS AT SIXTY

LIFE BEGINS AT SIXTY

BILL CASE

STEIN AND DAY/*Publishers*/New York

First published in 1986
Copyright © 1986 by Theodore W. Case
All rights reserved, Stein and Day, Incorporated
Designed by Louis A. Ditizio
Printed in the United States of America
STEIN AND DAY/*Publishers*
Scarborough House
Briarcliff Manor, N.Y. 10510

Library of Congress Cataloging-in-Publication Data

Case, Bill.
  Life begins at sixty.

  1. Retirement—United States. 2. Old age-United States—Psychological aspects. I. Title.
HQ1062.C38   1986   305.2′6   85-40719
ISBN 0-8128-3023-7

For Violet

CONTENTS

1. When Life Begins   9
2. Retirement Shock   19
3. Retirement to What?   35
4. Life Expectancy   45
5. To What Purpose?   57
6. Doing Good   69
7. Winds of Change   85
8. Variety   101
9. Hanging in There   113
10. The Man Who Did Everything   125
11. Sex After Sixty   145
12. Power   149
13. Keep Moving   167
14. Enjoy   181

APPENDIX: Some Organizations Whose Purpose Is to Assist Older Americans and Canadians   187

1

When Life Begins

> He lives long that lives well.
> —Thomas Fuller

"Life begins at sixty!" Nonsense. How can anybody say such a thing when clearly you have to have already lived for sixty years to have a sixtieth birthday? Fair enough, I guess, but if you want to rule out sixty, then when would you say life really does begin?

Does it begin at zero, the actual moment of birth? Or should zero really be taken to mean the moment of conception, which I believe is how the Chinese calculate it?

There is a lot to be said for the instant the wriggling sperm finally penetrates the egg. Yet one has to admit that the sperm and the egg each possessed life before their fateful rendezvous. Certainly each gene, with all its chromosomes, goes back a long, long way. Thinking about that feels like looking in a mirror that reflects me in another mirror, and yet another, with infinite me's going back into eternity.

Personally, I believe that life begins when I first open my eyes every morning. Something like a watch you wind every day. So maybe you can go along with me when I say, "Life begins at sixty or seventy or whenever you become determined enough to say it should." And in that regard, I will make you a promise right now. If you will read and think about the many people who are the subjects of each chapter in this book, your life will begin, whatever your chronological age, in a way you wouldn't have thought possible yesterday. The reason I chose sixty is because thereabouts is when life begins to end for all too many people. Oh, they may still be walking around, but they're not really living.

When I opened my eyes this morning, it was to find the sun flooding the room, the temperature at about 6 degrees, and one of those crystal clear, blue sky days that God sometimes gives New England in January, the day after a snowstorm. I thought about a cup of coffee and, perhaps, some toast with marmalade. And I thought about my purpose for this day: to start writing the first chapter of this book. There's nothing like a beginning to make one feel good. I happen to be 65 right now, but I am starting something new, and that gives this day, this month, and, yes, this year a shining cloak of adventure. No doubt about it, there can be newness and adventure anytime in your life. But we don't often get these good things by dreaming. How do we?

I've talked to hundreds of people during the writing of this book, and I've seen that those who live long lives, filled with vitality and joy, seem to have certain things in common. And they don't appear to be negative things such as not staying up too late, not drinking, not overdoing sex, not getting angry, not eating too much, not living under pressure, and other things of that nature. What they seem to have in common are positive things. They laugh a lot, they enjoy sex, they like variety, they live in places that stimulate them, they know what their powers are, and they enjoy exercising their power. Turn back a couple of pages and look at the table of contents. These are the areas the people I'm talking about know how to handle. Now, in the 1980s, those of us who want to enjoy our days after sixty, at least as much and possibly more than our earlier days, have a great many advantages that I think you'll recognize and agree with as you read further.

Of course I have used the scientific method throughout. We'll observe the way people behave, and then we'll draw our conclusions. The following example of a learned man using the scientific method

When Life Begins

might be helpful. He had trained a flea to jump over a matchstick whenever he said "jump." Notebook at his side, the scientist removed two of the flea's legs and then said, "Jump." Over the stick the flea went. He made a notation and then removed two more of the flea's six legs. "Jump," he said. Jump the flea did. After another scribble in the notebook, he removed the animal's last pair of legs. "Jump," he cried. Nothing. Now the scientist made the conclusive entry in his book: "When a flea loses all six legs," he wrote, "it becomes deaf." With that caveat on the scientific method, let's make some observations on the behavior of a sixty-year-old man.

It was back in the summer of 1934. Remember where you were that summer—and how old? The man we're observing was sixty. He sank a trowel in some wet cement, swirled it around, and lifted out a goodly glob, which he slapped down with gusto and smoothed out as he commenced laying another course of bricks. Some forty-five miles south of London, in the scented summer countryside, this apparently retired country gentleman was amusing himself building a handsome brick wall, improving both the privacy and beauty of his delightful garden.

If you watched closely you would notice that he seemed now and then to mumble and occasionally snort to himself. The cause of these volcanic rumblings was one Adolf Hitler who had just grasped full power across the Channel in Germany and was, even then, swaggering at the funeral of former President Hindenburg. But his major fulminations were not aimed at the rising Nazi power but, rather, at a myopic aristocracy and foolish British government that insisted "this Hitler was no more than an ill-bred clown"—certainly no threat to the government of George V, by the Grace of God, of Great Britain, Ireland, and the British Dominions beyond the seas, King, Defender of the Faith, Emperor of India, and so forth. No, our man was angry partly at the events but mostly at the fact of his inability to pursue his lifelong purpose of maintaining that empire.

Certainly, he could never have guessed that within five years a staggering Britain would turn to him for help and that by May 1940 he would be handed the seemingly hopeless task of turning back one

LIFE BEGINS AT SIXTY

relentless German assault after another. In fact, as England's leader, he would face the Nazi enemy virtually alone for two more long years before American help began to make itself felt.

As the shadows lengthen we observe him putting down his tools, surveying his work with satisfaction, and walking toward the house and, no doubt, a few brandies with his beloved wife, Clementine. He could look back on a long life of adventure and service to his country. It had begun in 1895 when he served with Spanish forces in Cuba. He was with British troops in India in 1897, and in Africa in 1898-99 during the Boer War, where he was taken prisoner and later escaped. He had been First Lord of the Admiralty during the first part of World War I and had held important posts in government after that war.

Now, in 1940, at the age of sixty-six, when most men have retired from the battles of life, Winston Churchill was only beginning the greatest battles of his life—activities in which his decisions and fierce determination would have important impact on the lives of millions around the globe. Sure, in a very real sense, his life was beginning at sixty-six. Thirteen years later, victory behind him, after three books and his six-volume *The Second World War,* he was awarded the Nobel Prize in literature—a nice seventy-ninth birthday present. When he died in 1965, at the age of 90, the world was quick to recognize him as one of the few who had exerted the greatest influence on the twentieth century.

"Well," I can hear you saying right now, "I'm not Winston Churchill. If I'd had his family background, his money, or his whatever . . ." Yes, I know, but remember our scientist and the flea and don't draw false conclusions from the example. The fact is that Churchill put on his pants one leg at a time, too. Perhaps the following story about the famous Jewish philosopher, Martin Buber, will make my point. He was discussing with a friend the measurement of a man's accomplishments during his lifetime. "You know," he said to his friend, "when the day of judgment comes, God is not going to ask me 'Why weren't you Moses?' He will ask me, 'Why weren't you Buber?'"

So don't worry about not being Winston Churchill, worry about not being . . . well, you know your name better than I do. It's what we

When Life Begins

have in common with Churchill that I want you to think about—the joy and zest he found in living, the fun and satisfaction he got out of painting and building his walls, his lively sense of humor, and his habit of constantly setting new goals for himself. Even in retirement—and the British people retired him over and over quite against his will—he immediately set out to do something, write a book, paint a picture, build another wall, or get reelected. He believed in laughter. Of Sir Stafford Cripps, a very dour Labour party minister, he said, "There, but for the grace of God, goes God." His outrageous statements got by because they were funny. When he was in power he used it without hesitation, and when he used it, he enjoyed it. So should you.

It seems very clear that there are certain elements that, when present in a person's life, cause that person to live a longer life and a life full of the pleasures, accomplishments, and just plain fun that make them glad to be alive at seventy-six, eighty-seven, or ninety-one. Well, those very elements are what this book is about. I've observed them in friends, in my grandmother, and in many other perfectly ordinary individuals.

I saw a woman close to ninety on TV the other night, suddenly, for a moment, take on the appearance of a twenty-year-old. The television show was a documentary about older people living in the mountains of rural Georgia. The interviewer was talking with a group around a fire at night and learned that two of them had been married sixty years. "How does it feel," he asked the man, "after being married that long?" "Sweeter and sweeter," replied the man, without a second's hesitation and with a glowing smile on his face. He looked like a happy man, but the face that really struck me was toward the side of the screen, that of his wife. I will never forget the sudden smile that illuminated that beautiful face. There, for a fleeting moment, I saw the twenty-year-old just as he must have seen her sixty years before. I think she was blushing, too.

Is it modern medicine that makes it possible for a Churchill, the old couple I just described, or someone like the famous American painter, Georgia O'Keefe, to accomplish so much into advanced age? Of course modern medicine has a great deal to do with all of us living longer and feeling better. I had a triple coronary bypass operation twelve years ago; and without that procedure I probably wouldn't be pecking away at this typewriter today.

On the other hand the state of medicine in Italy in 1547 had little to do with the ability of Michaelangelo to take over as chief architect of St. Peter's Cathedral in Rome at the age of 72 and to design and supervise construction for the next six years. And back in the twelfth century the beautiful Eleanor of Aquitaine, Queen of France and then of England, was a fury of political activity until her eighty-third year. And Benjamin Franklin, as American ambassador to France, was still fighting diplomatic battles in Paris for American independence at seventy-nine. Five years later, in his eighty-fifth year, he was active enough to be among the first to work in Congress for the abolition of slavery—although, unfortunately, it was an idea whose time had not yet come.

Looking at the thousands of human beings throughout history who have lived to a ripe old age, and continued to accomplish great things, you've got to admit there must have been something more than medicine involved. I think I have observed certain "life principles" that have been common to the lives of outstanding achievers throughout history. What follows is a combination of the best recommendations modern science can make and a discovery of those principles that appear to have operated throughout history in men and women who have lived long and lived well.

Dr. Erdman Palmore, of the Duke University Medical Center, has developed a longevity quotient for people over sixty based on a number of proveable and significant factors. I was interested to find that two of the major factors are "work satisfaction" and "happiness." The admonition "Enjoy!" is right on the mark, apparently.

One who would certainly second Dr. Palmore's conclusions is Norman Cousins, former publisher of *The Saturday Review of Literature,* and author of a book on his own extraordinary recovery from a serious illness. "Defeatism invites defeat," he writes. Hope, love, and laughter are the medicines he recommends for prolonging life.

A notion known as the "cosmic clock" has also surfaced recently. It

When Life Begins

suggests that there may be some kind of timing device built right into our cells that determines when their physical functions will wear out—unless an accident occurs earlier. Don't worry about the sinister ticking of that clock. If it does exist, the point at which the alarm goes off is many years beyond the point most humans reach, as you will see in the chapter on "life expectancy."

Perhaps the most convincing aspect of Professor Palmore's work is the fact that he checked his conclusions about the same group fifteen years later. He had been looking for a single observation about his group that could predict long life and his choice had been "work satisfaction... as the best predictor." When he checked the group after fifteen years, he found that his best predictions were thirty-three percent more accurate than those based on ordinary actuarial life expectancy. The word that jumps out at me is "satisfaction." Think of the need to have fun, the need for variety, the need to do good, and the need for action. Those needs need satisfying, and if we go on for very long without the pleasure of their satisfaction, life becomes a bore at best.

It appears to me that life, for most people, divides itself roughly into three segments: zero to thirty years of age, thirty to sixty, and sixty to ninety-plus. The activities of most of us in these periods seem able to be characterized thus: zero to thirty, LEARNING; thirty to sixty, EARNING; and sixty to ninety-plus... well, what should we call that? The word that keeps coming into my head is LIVING. It's exactly what I believe. Beginning at sixty, yes, those are the great years for living—and an awful lot of people are missing out on it.

LEARNING, we now know, begins even before birth. The fetus is already reacting to stimuli and developing behaviorial action patterns that can be characterized as rudimental learning. For some people such as doctors and other highly specialized professionals, the formal learning period extends beyond the age of thirty. What is happening in this period is that human knowledge, painfully gained over thousands of years, is being acquired for use in the lifetime that follows. This process should never end. If it does, reading this book would be a waste of your time.

EARNING, of course, often begins well before thirty, but during the second thirty years is when the most significant earning takes place. "In the sweat of thy face" as we read in the Old Testament, and there can be no escaping working and earning. Frankly, I'd hate to think of those thirty years of my life as empty of achievement. Oh, sea and sun, endless pleasure, empty days . . . they may seem to beckon when we drag ourselves home after a punishing day's work, but, translated into reality, they add up to nothing less than early death—of the mind, of the competitive spirit, of the thrill of winning, and the satisfaction of accomplishment. No, these are great years, and for most, they can last well beyond sixty. But whenever the "earning" period ends, we of the magic twentieth century find ahead of us a period mankind as a whole has never known before.

As recently as the beginning of this century, the number of people who lived beyond the age of sixty was not that great. Figuring out what to do with those years was no problem. Today that third segment of our lives offers us the opportunity to simply enjoy living.

Think for a moment about the view from sixty. Ahead lie twenty or thirty or even more years; years that have possibly more potential for enjoyment and achievement than any in the past. Until this point, for most of us, circumstances have molded our decisions, have subtly guided us, sometimes forced our lives into channels that may not have been our first choice. For the great majority, those middle years have been a series of compromises—distortions of our dreams if not abandonment of them. Pressures from both known and unexpected sources have pulled and hauled at our lives until the actual zigzag course bore little resemblance to what we had planned at twenty.

Love is the greatest thing, no doubt about that; but it does have certain sobering consequences. Children are a common result. It becomes necessary to rent or buy a home, which calls for untold sums of money. Fortunately, your friendly banker was ready to advance the many thousands of dollars, all the while twirling his mustache, which it took most of your working life to repay. A car or cars become necessary, also available through the simple act of putting your signature on a piece of paper. Thus, most of us were required to produce large sums of money every month, which had a firm effect on

When Life Begins

how we spent our working hours and days. Eventually, a few decades later, we found that our salaries had grown respectably, our financial lives had smoothed somewhat, and we started taking real vacations once in a while. Enter the ax, falling. Some of our children wanted to go to college. All of our children wanted to go to college. *We* wanted all of our children to go to college. Or a daughter wanted to get married—in church. Get out pencil and paper or, today, switch on the home computer. And a few more decisions had been made for us.

Well, now we have arrived at sixty, battered, somewhat bloody, but, we hope, unbowed. And it's the view from sixty I want you to think about as you emerge, disoriented and still shaken from those EARNING years. For some, it's a time for retirement; others have already retired; and some are planning for it. A few wouldn't think of it. But for virtually all, the pressure is off! Our lives have suddenly become our own! Of course, there will always be things we want to do for our children, but the hard pressure of having to provide this or that is lifted. The feeling can be giddy, as if, emerging from a long tunnel, we find ourselves blinded by the light.

Those who have planned moderately well will find they have income from a number of sources: social security, a pension from the organization they worked for, some income from investments, and so on. And as most survey their coming sixties, seventies, and eighties, their attitude is usually one of bewilderment. What is going to happen? they think. How long will I live? What shall I do? Is it going to be fun? or awful?

We're told today, by the "professionals," that children and teenagers need the right role models so they'll avoid drugs and crime and lead decent lives. The pages that follow are full of role models for us children in our sixties. I want you to meet the people in this book and think about their lives, because it seems to me that the example of vitality in other human lives influences us and sets our blood moving in a manner that abstract theorizing never could. We are never separate from the efforts and successes and simple human happinesses of other people. What they do is waiting for us; what they *can* do, we, in our way, can do also.

2

Retirement Shock

Rest is rust.
—William H. Seward

"Withdraw, depart, leave, retreat." These words are all synonyms for the subject of this chapter: "retirement." They don't, especially the last one, seem like very good things to do. Yet most businesses and our governments have selected arbitrary dates when they force us to "retreat," or whichever synonym you prefer. They throw parties, give us presents, make happy speeches, and in general, celebrate the occasion. Yet I have always detected sinister, almost funereal, undercurrents at such occasions.

"He's going, we're staying."

"He really *was* a great guy."

Was already? And almost everyone says, "Well, what are you going to do now, Sam?" One of the best answers is always, "We've bought a camper, and we're going to see the good old U.S.A. at last. Never had the time before." Or, in more rarified circles, "We've planned a slow trip around the world—there's an awful lot to see out there." You could probably just as easily say, "We're blasting off for the moon right after the next neap tide. Planning a couple of weeks on the Sea of Tranquility," and you'd get the same glass-eyed stare in response. The

LIFE BEGINS AT SIXTY

fact is, you're already gone as far as they're concerned. And if you're not careful, you may really be gone within the next twelve months.

Diseases of the circulatory system and cancer are named today as the major causes of passing on to whatever comes next. Yet a pretty good number of wise heads place another event, "retirement," at the top of that list. How often, how very, very often, do we hear: "And he just retired less than a year ago"? "Much too young to die, really." The connection between the two events is all too real in many cases; but we know, too, of the many exceptions, those who charge right on for twenty or thirty more years—or even *lope* right on for many more happy years.

The devastating shock of retirement after thirty or forty years is really known only to those who experience it. The sudden switch from a highly structured environment where one has a definite place and an acknowledged status to a void where one becomes, to a great extent, "Who?", batters both the mental and physical being. The retiring president is no longer greeted by the doorman, receptionist, secretaries, junior executives, and vice-presidents at the start of every day. He no longer has to juggle his business lunches during the week; no more is he rushed to Kennedy in a limo, lifted magically in a 747 to Heathrow, London, and deposited at the Inn on the Park by another limo; people don't even stand when he enters the room anymore; mail is no longer a problem; and his telephone stops ringing. His telephone stops ringing, "ay, there's the rub." Nobody needs him anymore.

His name is John. He's run the mailroom for more years than anyone can remember. From the chairman to the snippiest secretary, he has a certain standing. He *is* the U.S. Postal Service, Emery Air Freight or Federal Express—even United Parcel Service. And in addition to the postage meter, he's got wrapping paper and tape! It's Christmas: "John, this is for my niece, and I've left it too late. Do you think you could possibly wrap it for me and maybe get it out today." Or "John, my mother's birthday is next Tuesday, and I completely forgot it. Do you think you could possibly . . . ?" Or the president's executive secretary drops into the mail room, "John, Mr. Steele wants one of those big stamping machines in Chicago by noon tomorrow—and it isn't even crated. Do you think . . . ?"

Then they give John a party, a watch, and the pension paperwork, and the following week his wife is saying, "John, would you please stay out of the kitchen? You just don't know where anything goes, and it's easier for me to do things my way." Suddenly nobody "needs John anymore." Oh, there are those who love him, those who like him, even those who admire him—but who *needs* John now?

I know of no more wonderful feeling than when somebody lets me know they need me. Wife, granddaughter, son, son-in-law—when one of them unwittingly lets me know they need me for something specific, I swell with pride, purpose, and the knowledge that I am good for something. I said "unwittingly" because I don't particularly hunger for someone to say "I need you" anymore than I want my wife to say "I love you" daily. What I want is for her to *love* me, not to *say* she loves me.

So the newly liberated individual, no matter what his or her position in the business profession or whatnot, is struck by "retirement shock." He wakes up the morning after to find himself in a vacuum, with no position, no particular function, no sycophants, and nobody who even wants to weasel something out of him. Retirement shock can be fatal. It very often is unless you do something about it *yesterday*. "Yesterday" is the operative word because shockless retirement is usually the result of preparation and planning.

I hope I'm not giving the impression that retirement is equivalent to a sentence of death. There are a great many people who sweep past that sixty- or sixty-five-year milestone with hardly a glance and go on into their eighties and nineties living the fullest and richest of lives. Some of them never retire, that is, retreat from what they have been doing all their lives. Others fall back (in the military sense) only to regroup and attack life on another front. I'd like to list a few of these people.

There are instructions for reading this list. Pay attention and do it

LIFE BEGINS AT SIXTY

like this: *Do not* compare yourself to the people whose names follow. Instead try to *relate* to them. "What the hell does that mean?" I can hear you thinking. I mean try to empathize with them; try to understand their motives. Look for something in yourself that is similar to them—maybe a latent ambition, a dream you hardly dare admit, possibly a vague attitude you share with all of them or some of them. The first group is made up of famous people—the majority of them dead. The second group (not so famous) is doing fine, and most are alive, thank you. Both groups have at least two things in common: They lived very long lives. They lived or are living very rich lives. And that's what *Life Begins at Sixty* is about.

Socrates—First a sculptor, then a philosopher. Developed a method of teaching by questioning, leading students to reach rational conclusions. Continued until the age of seventy-one, when he was forced to drink hemlock.

Plato—Student of Socrates and teacher of Aristotle; philosopher and founder of history's first university. Prolific writer until his death at 82.

Sophocles—Greek dramatist, born 496 B.C., one of the three greatest Greek playwrights. He was also a general and imperial treasurer. Wrote 123 plays, of which seven survive and are still regularly performed. Finished his last play, *Oedipus at Colonus* just before his death at ninety.

Elizabeth Cady Stanton—Fighter for women's rights. Organized first women's rights convention in 1848. Effected introduction to U.S. Congress the amendment to the Constitution that granted women's suffrage and that finally passed after her death in 1921. Was working on this bill when she died at eighty-six.

Helena Rubenstein—One of America's most successful businesswomen. Established company that she built, then shrewdly sold in 1929—buying it back at enormous profit two years later. In the thirty-five years following her sixtieth birthday, she built Helena

Rubenstein into the most successful cosmetics company in the world.
Pablo Picasso—Spanish painter and sculptor; one of two or three greatest influences on art world in the twentieth century. Fathered two children in his sixties; created works of art until the age of ninety-one.
Claude Pepper—Member of U.S. Congress since 1930s. Heavily influenced by FDR; has dedicated his life to service of people. Understands the system, uses of power, and how to get things done—and still does so at eighty-five, particularly for the benefit of older Americans.
Gloria Swanson—American actress whose career spanned the history of film, silent and sound. Retired before World War II; during war, formed business manufacturing luminous paint. Came back to movies in *Sunset Boulevard*; took up painting and held successful show in London in 1978. Continued living vigorously until her death at 84.
Michelangelo—Italian painter, sculptor, architect, and poet. Produced an incredible volume of the highest rank of work from his youth until the age of 89, when he was working on plans for the transformation of the Baths of Diocletian into a church and on new fortifications for Rome.
Armand Hammer—Self-made oil tycoon (Occidental Petroleum Corporation). International negotiator for peace on his own initiative; now, at eighty-six, he bounces on his private jet to his homes in New York, Canada, Moscow, London, and California, making his own efforts, not without impact, to lessen differences between the East and West.

HAD ENOUGH OF famous oldsters through the ages? I could extend the list for pages. I haven't even mentioned such names as Ronald Reagan, George Burns, George Bernard Shaw, Sir John Gielgud, or Jacques Cousteau. I could have talked about the Italian Renaissance painter Titian, who was painting in his nineties; or the Spanish painter Goya; or the Italian composer Verdi, who wrote his last great opera, *Falstaff*, when he was eighty. But I feel sure a few points have been made. Living gloriously into the seventies, eighties, or nineties is not a new phenomenon; people have been doing it for thousands of years. Man's life span was meant to be, and probably always has been, potentially, near one hundred years.

Now, I'm going to ask you to look at a few more minibiographies; this time they will be of people who did not make the history books or "Who's Who" but who are our contemporaries.

Bernard Splaver—Bridgeport, Connecticut. Retired caterer. After retirement, joined faculty and became dean of the Culinary Institute of America. Retired again. Now very active in SCORE (Service Corps of Retired Executives), giving advice and active assistance to young businessmen. Splaver is eighty-six.

Nancy Hopkins Tier—Member of the famous "Ninety-Nines" first women's airplane pilot group; vice-president of the newly completed Women's Air and Space Museum in Dayton, Ohio. Now 76, Mrs. Tier is celebrating 58 years as a pilot, regularly flying her Cessna 170A for business and pleasure throughout the United States and Canada.

Elizabeth Cotten—Guitarist, folk music singer and composer, she wrote her first song, "Freight Train," when eleven years old. She grew up with music from her parents and grandparents (the latter freed slaves), earned $3.75 for her first guitar at nine, and now, at ninety, she continues to concertize in New York, Washington, and around the country.

Berenice Abott—Blanchard, Maine. Photographer who captured Hemingway, Scott Fitzgerald, and other to-be-famous expatriate American artists and writers in Paris in the twenties. Still an active professional photographer at eighty-four, Mrs. Abott is starting piano lessons and remains one of the better table tennis players in Blanchard.

Lina Basquette—Wheeling, West Virginia. Former Ziegfeld Follies dancer in the twenties, a star in a Cecil B. deMille movie, Ms. Basquette retired at forty-one to raise Great Danes; and now, at seventy-eight, she is a professional show-dog handler.

Reynolds Wait—Auburn, New York. Owner-manager of string of furniture stores, he shunned retirement and drove twenty miles to work daily, until at 91, he decided to accept rides. Ran the stores himself until a few weeks before he died in 1976 at ninety-three.

Dr. Karel Steinbach—Recently retired as physician at the Brooklyn, New York, Fort Hamilton Induction Center, where he had processed all women applicants to the armed forces since 1965. At eighty-eight he felt that driving on Brooklyn-Queens highways on dark mornings was dangerous.

BOTH OF THESE lists of the famous and people just like ourselves could have been many times longer, but they will have served their purpose if your reaction is "My God, sixty years old is just a beginning." It certainly was for these people and it's doubtful that at their sixtieth birthdays they dreamed what was still to come.

And how did you do in relating to some of these oldsters? Sophocles, who lived some twenty-four hundred years ago, sounds like something of what we call a "workaholic" today. One hundred twenty-three plays is a lot to write even if he hadn't served as a general in two wars and been city treasurer. Are you that kind of "firecracker"? It doesn't seem to have done Sophocles any harm, and he surely kept busy. How about Ronald Reagan? He seems to have moved fairly smoothly from acting to politics within his union, then to state, and finally, national politics. And when you see him climb on his horse at his California ranch, he surely looks in good shape.

Of course when it comes to Titian or Sir John Gielgud or George Burns or Picasso, one can always say, "Well, if I'd been born that talented, of course I could live a long time and accomplish great things." It's a trap! Don't fall into it. I doubt that a great many readers will have heard of Bernard Splaver, of Bridgeport, or Reynolds Wait, of Auburn, both also very busy into their late eighties and early nineties, respectively. But you can't disassociate from them with the "born talented" line. The fact is that all these people just kept "a-chuggin,'" and while doing so, they lived and enjoyed life as they wanted.

And there's another common "out"; it goes like this: If people have great health and natural energy, then they live long, active, and happy lives. It might appear to be true but from what I've seen in researching this book, the facts are just the opposite. People who live active, happy, and fulfilled (to their way of thinking) lives tend to have better health than others. In fact, I see this phenomenon as an endless circle: Activity leads to health, leads to energy, leads to a rich life, leads to more of all these, and finally, leads to a long, fulfilled life. If there's a common thread among the lives of the people mentioned, it is this: **THEY NEVER RETIRED.** Of course, some of them retired several times but it was always to return to an activity that they cared for.

But, there are those, many unfortunately, who just can't handle retirement, who find themselves like a rudderless ship, drifting aimlessly, unable to get moving on any course. Usually they have given little or no thought to what will come the morning after the retirement party.

Let me give you an example. I'm not going to use the person's real name. We'll call him George. I guess the main reason for telling you about him is that his life, after retirement, lacks every one of those qualities that are required for living long and living well. I mean life qualities like *variety* or having *purpose* that are the subjects of the chapters to come and that you'll see illustrated in the lives of the people you'll be reading about.

Mary is a neighbor who has known George pretty well for a number of years. "George was very happy before he retired," she replied to my first question. "He worked with communications equipment for a large company. He was good at his job and proud of the way they'd always come to him when there was a particularly tough problem. 'Call George, he can do it,' that's what he liked to hear. But then, because of some merger or something, his work place was going to be moved to a town some sixty miles away. And he didn't like that."

"How old was he then?" I asked.

"He was sixty-three then," Mary said. "And he either had to move or drive some sixty miles to work and back every day. So he checked it out and found he could handle retirement financially. His Social

Retirement Shock

Security, his pension, and a little income from savings would take perfectly good care of George and his wife. So he took the plunge."

Everything went fine for the first six months. He had himself a wonderful time with his new-found freedom. He traveled around visiting all his children, seeing a new grandchild, and just enjoying himself. Then everything changed.

"Boy, I'll tell you, suddenly, it was like overnight," Mary said, "just like overnight." He wasn't happy anymore. He had no purpose. He had seen everything he wanted to see in the region where they lived. He had come to some sort of an end.

"And it came without any warning," Mary said. "They could have done anything—gone to Europe—Hawaii. And now all of a sudden money became a great problem."

"A real problem?" I asked.

"No, not at all," she said. "But he claimed it was. He just started going into a shell. He got paranoid that his money was going to run out. You know what I think hit him? I think what hit him was 'I'm not working to earn this money anymore—and I couldn't make any more if I wanted to.' The fixed income paralyzed him."

He started doing very strange things such as putting his money in a lot of different banks. At the same time, he began exhibiting odd behavior in other parts of his life. One day he went to the "Goodwill" shop and bought a jacket for three dollars. And yet on the very next day he went to a shoe store and paid ninety dollars for a pair of shoes he didn't need. His behavior in general became highly inconsistent.

"One night," Mary said, "he became very irritated with his wife because she had bought a beef roast for dinner. She should have bought bologna. Yet just a few days later, when his wife did buy bologna, he complained just as loudly that she should have bought roast beef. And so his life at home deteriorated, and he gradually became a complete loner. He would still walk downtown occasionally to the barber shop to chat with the barber whom he'd known for years. But even then most of what he had to say was fault-finding, complaining about the world today and how everything was 'going to pot.'

LIFE BEGINS AT SIXTY

"Now he doesn't even do that much," Mary went on. "He sleeps a great deal of the time, not just naps—it seems he is really trying to kill time."

"How's his health?" I asked Mary.

"Perfect, just perfect. The doctor says it's perfect. But, to hear him—he thinks he's got everything—something new all the time. He'll say he's tired, there must be something wrong with his blood-sugar level, and so on, and so on.

"But mostly, he's just wasting his time away. And he's taken to doing some of the most ridiculous things. Here's a man who has—or had—absolutely no sense of humor. Now, he's suddenly taken to visiting the stationery shops just to read the funny greeting cards. He does it like going to the library. And then, he'll buy the cards—not to send to anyone—just to show them to people to laugh at."

But one of the things that worries Mary most is the way George is becoming more and more isolated—from his wife, from his friends, and from society at large. Before, he used to get up in the morning and do something—perhaps take a little drive or drop in on a friend—now, he's taken to sleeping later and later. "It's from bed to his rocking chair and the TV and back to bed," is how Mary describes it.

Mary says he is becoming more and more withdrawn. "He'll watch television for hours, with the sound turned off. We're all just worried to death about what will happen next," she concluded.

I don't know how George's situation will finally resolve itself, but I wanted you to see an example that illustrates a complete lack of all those life qualities that lead to happy retirements and rich and contented years after sixty.

LET'S CONSIDER A few cases of people who thumbed their noses at the very idea of retirement. Take Martie Tafel whose motto might be, "Who says you can't fight city hall?" He not only fought it, but he went right on to tilt with the windmills at the state capitol. Marten Tafel has been a science teacher many years in the Westport, Connecticut, school system. And as most of us over sixty know, federal law has raised the mandatory retirement age to seventy. Of course, when an employer is agreeable there's nothing to stop someone staying on in his job; but when Tafel reached that age of seventy, he was informed that the state required his retirement from teaching.

Steeped in the scientific method as he was, Tafel decided to examine the facts and reach his own conclusions. He has never been a man to ask "How high?" when told to jump! He dug up the state statutes on retirement and looked for himself. The law did call for retirement at seventy. Here is how he told it to me.

"I noticed, however, that it read, 'A teacher may be retained under certain conditions.' I reread the fool thing carefully and I said, 'Oh, I know what *may* means—it's not *shall* or *must*, it means *may*. So I went to the A.C.L.U. and said, 'How about that?' But they said, 'No.' Apparently, like the Lord, their eye was on the sparrow—at least the A.C.L.U. was certainly not watching me.

"Then I went to my union," he continued. "I believe in unions, and I've always belonged to the Connecticut Education Association. I went up there and they said, 'We can't do anything about that, there isn't any ground swell.' I said what do you mean, no ground swell. There *is* a ground swell of seventy-year-old people! And I ranted and I raved and said, 'All these years, you haven't done a goddamned thing for me up to now. And here I'm asking you.' Nothing.

"So I did the only thing left to me, I hired a local law firm. They thought we ought to sue the board of education. But they weren't against me. In fact they wanted to help me. It turned out that it was the state we had to go after. So I have to tell you it was poetic justice. On my seventieth birthday papers were served on Ella Grasso (then governor), the attorney general, and all the other assorted functionaries involved.

"Well, I'm happy to tell you that the attorney general had to sit down and carefully reread that statute. And he found that word 'may' just as I had. The upshot was that he did a little rewriting just to clarify the whole thing, and I'm proud to tell you that today there are seventeen people over seventy teaching in Connecticut schools."

It made me proud of my age group to hear Martie Tafel tell his story and to hear the vigor and determination that permeated his voice. Now, however, at seventy-seven he really has retired.

"Then, what are you doing now?" I asked him.

"Well, the first day I did three loads of laundry. The second day I did the windows and floors. On the third day I went to Washington for a meeting of the National Science Teachers Association. I blush to tell you that last year I received a citation for distinguished service from that association. I got back here last night, and Tuesday I'll be leaving for Cape Hatteras for a meeting of an oceanology group I belong to. We'll be meeting at William and Mary for a couple of days, then spend some time on Chesapeake Bay, and, finally, down to Cape Hatteras for some surf casting—about which I know nothing. The only way I'll catch anything is if the fish swims ashore and commits suicide!"

I believe the present law that permits companies to mandate retirement at seventy will probably bite the dust in the near future. I certainly hope it does because it has very little relation to reality.

HERE'S ANOTHER SEPTUAGENARIAN who resisted the retirement statute and, with the help of an even less orthodox approach, made it to eighty-one. We'll call him Hal.

"At age seventy-three," Hal said, "I voluntarily retired." But he reports that the following year turned out to be one of frustrating idleness. "Found I was just going nuts," is the way he put it. "My background is sales, management, and advertising, and I knew I was fully capable both mentally and physically. Yet, no matter what I tried, I was regularly turned down because of my age.

"Feeling really desperate, I revised my résumé—in one respect only—I took eleven years off my age. In less than two months I had a good job—a job that incidentally I held for the next seven years. Then, once again, I reached the mandatory retirement age of 'seventy' and was forced to retire. In reality, of course, I was then eighty-one—and, I might add, just as able both mentally and physically as when they hired me."

I must admit that the way in which Hal handled his age problem, or

Retirement Shock

rather *other people's* problem with his age, makes a beautiful case for retirement based on performance rather than on a number that has a different meaning for every individual to whom it is applied.

FOR A REALLY dramatic contrast, consider a lady who until recently did three shows a day on television at the mature age of ninety. Dorothy Fuldheim was a foreign correspondent and editorial commentator for WSEW-TV, Cleveland, for thirty-six years, and she was given virtually carte blanche to go anywhere in the world for a story. This freedom took her to Hong Kong, Northern Ireland, Germany, Egypt, Australia, England, and a dozen other exotic places.

Fuldheim got her start as a speaker and editorializer with a push from Jane Addams, a major figure in social settlement work in the United States and the founder of Hull House in Chicago. Fuldheim had started as an actress, and in 1913 Addams saw her in the play *The State Forbids* and urged her to take up public speaking. "Thanks to Jane Addams," Fuldheim says, "I tried a lecture in Philadelphia a year later. Somebody said I'd done a good job, and I supported myself and my family on lecturing for a long time." In fact, she continued lecturing for more than thirty years until the daily television commitment interfered. Widowed twice, she has a crippled granddaughter who provides one reason for her will to secure a raise and continue working. "I've never been rich, never accepted aid from anyone, but I lost my daughter when she was thirty-eight of heart disease. She was beautiful, had earned a Ph.D., had a delightful sense of humor, and was very courageous. Now, I want to be sure my granddaughter has enough when I die."

When we spoke of age, Fuldheim just said, "Well, I don't know what all the fuss is about. So I'm going to be ninety." She had received attention from all over the world on the occasion. But she put forward an interesting hypothesis to me. "I think evolution is going on," she suggested. "For example, I think there are two manifestations of evolution: one is living longer, the other is the expansion of the brain. How else can you explain the bold thinking that is taking place today? I think maybe I'm one of the evolutionary species."

LIFE BEGINS AT SIXTY

I, perhaps unkindly, mentioned Sophocles, who died in 406 B.C. after finishing his 123d play at the age of ninety. "Well," she replied spiritedly, "He didn't get *his* contract renewed, you know." A strain of vigorous competitiveness showed there that may provide something of a clue to the lady's long and vigorous career. As far as her durability goes, I think the following airplane propeller incident provides incontrovertible evidence. As a pilot since 1937, I have never heard of anybody who survived walking into a spinning prop. "It happened in 1938," Fuldheim said. "I had just come back from Germany—it was in Akron, Ohio—and I was walking toward a friend's airplane and I just walked into the spinning propeller. It was made of wood—I don't know if that made the difference. I was hit on the arm and shoulder, and I actually walked for a while and then fell down. Later, my breasts were all black-and-blue. Of course, they got me on a stretcher right away. I thought at the time that there must be—I don't know—that destiny had not marked me." That acceptance of whatever life deals out is typical of the people in this book. If it is an attitude that can be cultivated; I highly recommend it. I know I could use more of it myself. Perhaps—when I get a little older . . .

Fuldheim told me that in her television career she had interviewed just about everybody. "Back in the thirties I met both Hitler and Mussolini. But for them, I was undesirable because I was one of the first people—I said that Hitler would bring Europe down, and I also said that Mussolini would help—and of course, Mussolini didn't like that. But you know, I wasn't farsighted. You could see it—it was there."

She returned to Germany in the 1960s to interview Albert Speer, Hitler's minister of armaments and war production. She relived the moment, "I got the story firsthand from him about how Hitler died. Extraordinary story. Speer was in the bunker, and he was at the wedding of Hitler and Eva Braun the day before they committed suicide. He also told me about Goebbels and how he had his five children killed before himself and his wife."

Talking with Speer, she said she found it difficult to believe that a seemingly gentle and cultivated man could have done what he did. But when she asked him, he said, "I had sold myself to ambition because Hitler offered me the opportunity to rebuild Berlin as Haussmann had rebuilt Paris." Speer was an architect and, according to Fuldheim, he added, "Once I took it [the opportunity], I would have been killed by Hitler if I tried to back out. He'd have hung me on a hook like a dead cow."

"Well, it would have been a worthy death, wouldn't it?" Fuldheim boldly replied.

WHY AM I going on about these people who have lived or are now living, to busy, enjoyable old age? It comes out of the research I've been doing, out of getting to know these people. Lately, I've noticed a distinct change in my own attitude toward age. When I started I thought of sixty as getting old, seventy as pretty old, and eighty as even older, and ninety—well, ninety was really over the hill. Now I'm surprised to find in myself quite a new perception of this third period of life that in the last chapter I called the LIVING years. Sixty is now young, a beginning. Seventy is when a lot of people are really just getting started. Eighty is a burgeoning, active middle age. Ninety, well that's still getting on a bit, but not apparently for the likes of Dorothy Fuldheim.

3

Retirement to What?

> You are hale, Father William—a hearty old man:
> Now tell me the reason, I pray.
> —Robert Southey

Dorothy Fuldheim did not choose to retire, and fortunately, for her, the organization she works for went along with that decision. Many of us are not offered that option. What to do if you're not ready to leave the work scene? Something near twenty years, more or less, lies ahead of us, and this may well be the greatest challenge and opportunity of a lifetime. You've seen what is happening with George, who appears to be slipping into a kind of paralysis. One thing is clearly lacking in George's life, something so important that later on I am going to devote an entire chapter to it. That element, without which life becomes little more than a treadmill, is purpose.

Nobody should drop out of life at sixty or sixty-five—at a time, if ever there was one, to begin. Now's the time to look around. What haven't you done yet in life? What have you always wanted to do and have put off so long you may have actually forgotten it? What are the opportunities waiting for you? What's sitting out there just crying to be done? Let's assume that you're not the type to want to bury yourself in work again, to "tote that barge, lift that bale." It's a time for fun. It may be called anything from a hobby to an avocation to a second career. Activities range from stamp collecting to raising racing pigeons, to hybridizing flowers (developing new varieties), to writing a book, to becoming the all-time North American expert on trout fishing.

In fact, I know one man who took early retirement and set out to learn everything he could about fly fishing. Now, a few years later, Leon Ogrodnik, of Williamstown, Massachusetts, has assembled a library of more than five hundred books and literally thousands of magazines on the subject.

In Ogrodnik's library one is literally surrounded by the trappings of fishing. A lamp shade, for example, is decorated with more than fifty colorful flies, hooks pressed right through the material of the shade. Anything that is on hand is grist for Ogrodnik's fly-tying mill. He once admired the silky hair of the tail of my black-and-white Pekinese. A few strands were extracted, painlessly I hope for Pun-Kin, and a brand new lure was born. And of course, there is an elaborate collection of rods, modern and antique. Ogrodnik has more than fifty rods of all kinds.

I had expected to see mounted fish on every wall, but only two or three specimens were displayed. "The trend among fishermen today is toward 'catch and release,'" he said. "An exceptional fish may be kept for mounting—and of course, there are those caught for eating—but the practice is to return most to the water. There's a lot more to fishing than fish, you know. I have always found that fishing is something of a spiritual experience in that it brings you in contact with so much beauty not experienced from day to day."

Once one develops a lively interest in one area, it can be surprising where the initial interest leads. Once, while attending a meeting of between two and three hundred fly fishermen, Ogrodnik met a scientist whose field of interest was acid rain. This man had done a great deal of research on the effects of acid rain on the trout population of lakes and streams. Ogrodnik told me he asked the scientist what was being done about the situation, and the scientist told him they were trying to develop an acid-resistant trout. "I was truly staggered by the implications of that statement," Ogrodnik said. "It really opened up Pandora's box for me. Because what ran through all of our minds was, What about the forage base and the ecology of this system? All my life I had felt very comfortable and very secure in the out-of-doors world. Now, all of a sudden, I felt very vulnerable."

The upshot of that experience is that Ogrodnik has become a very vocal and effective force in the acid rain controversy raging in the Northeast and Canada. One thing does lead to another, and as you will see, these are the things that give life its vitality, its color, and even its value.

But an avocation or a hobby is not the only activity following retirement that can satisfy, and give meaning to, life. Some just take a year off and look the world over and then choose to start a new job or career, as Benny Townsend has done at seventy-four.

BENJAMIN TOWNSEND IS half Shinnecock Indian and half black. He grew up, as he describes it, as a waif in Westbury, Long Island. He was first taken care of by a "kind lady," Mrs. Margaret Willis, who finally died at the age of 102. Later, he was unofficially adopted by an Italian family who brought him to semiadulthood. In the ordinary sense of the word, he was neither rich nor talented nor privileged. A couple of years ago Townsend retired from a long career with American Airlines and Allied Aviation as a mechanic in both airframe and engine maintenance and construction. A year of idleness was enough for him. "I finally got tired of drinking and playing cards," is how he put it. So in the fall of 1982, Townsend became a taxicab driver, an occupation he enjoys thoroughly.

He's not an artist or writer; he's not an actor; he's not wealthy; he's not a talented comedian like George Burns. The only "special" thing about him is the way he looks at life and looks at himself. I defy anybody to say of Townsend, "Well, if only I had his this or his that, I'd be a great happy guy in my middle seventies, too." Yet he has something that makes him different from other seniors who have "dropped out." His interest in mechanics surfaced early when, at fifteen, he "took a Cadillac apart and put it back together again." This interest led to his joining American Airlines in 1939 and spending the next twenty years on engine maintenance. Later, he switched to Allied Aviation, a company servicing all the airlines. After mandatory retirement, he worked as a skycap at Newark Airport. Still later, he found employment with the U.S. Department of Agriculture. In the department he was responsible for dunning individuals in delinquency on mortgage payments. This job required that he use a word processor, a not inconsiderable skill for a man in his seventies to acquire. Without question Townsend is not only a jack-of-all-trades but also a master of most of them. His final retirement, which lasted less than a year, came after Agriculture. And now he still pushes his cab around Manhattan and to Kennedy and La Guardia. And it's no "cushy" job; he's on the streets by 4 A.M. and works until three in the afternoon five days a week.

But that's not the end of Townsend's day. He is a gardener in residence for the home he and his wife share with a retired beauty shop owner. "I've got a twenty-eight- to thirty-foot-long philodendron I've cultivated over the years," he says proudly. "I clip and trim two hundred feet of hedges, and I've got two dozen roses waiting to be planted right now." Asked when he found the time, he replied, "Between four and five to six o'clock at night, I'm a gardener. And I have the weekends." Like many men, Townsend has his club, the "Soul Gears" motorcycle club, where he often stays until eleven or twelve o'clock at night exchanging tall tales with the "boys." He also belongs to the local "Playboy" club. His interests are wide. For example, he recently attended a seminar on "Sexology" at Trenton State College. "It's really a different era today," he said. "The young ladies were laughing at things women my age were looking serious or shocked at."

"I take life as it comes," pretty well states his attitude. "I'm not concerned about tomorrow or the future." With crime the way it is today, I asked him if he ever worried about anything happening to

Retirement to What?

him in his cab. "No, I never worry," he said. "The only thing ever happened to me—I got carbon monoxide poisoning once. It was leaking into the cab. But I recognized it from the dry throat—that's a sign, you know. They had me on oxygen for four hours. Didn't bother me though."

However, there's one thing Townsend doesn't appear to accept. He says, "My wife's always saying, 'You don't think you're a senior citizen, do you?'" He laughed happily. "I feel beautiful—I love the way I feel."

SOMETIMES IT'S A little difficult to tell whether a person has really retired or not. Lina Basquette was a dancer by profession for many years; she quit that shortly after World War II, but is she retired now? Let me tell you about this lady who danced in 1915 at the San Francisco World's Fair, appeared in a silent film in the twenties, visited Adolf Hitler at his "Eagle's Nest" in the thirties, then entertained Allied soldiers during World War II. After the war she retired from professional dancing and started her own kennels to breed and raise Great Danes. In time, her kennels became the largest and most successful in the United States and Basquette went into professional show-dog handling. Now, in her late seventies, she shows dogs all over North America. I first saw her running a champion Great Dane around Madison Square Garden at the Westminster Kennel Club Show. If you've ever watched one of these events you'll know how fast the handler runs to show a little Yorkshire terrier at its best. To show a Great Dane to best advantage, you've got to do the hundred-yard dash in pretty good time. To show her dog, Special K-Gribbin, to win the dog's thirty-first best-of-group ribbon, this lady was as fleet-footed as you could want, and she's 78 years old. Not only did the dog win, but the handler got a rave review in a column in *The New York Times* the next day under the title, "A Ziegfeld Girl Keeps Running." When we were talking about it, she said to me, "How do you like that? I had to run a dog around Madison Square Garden to get a good review in *The New York Times.*"

Lina Basquette calculates she has driven more than a million miles

LIFE BEGINS AT SIXTY

from her home in Wheeling to show Great Danes. During the past two years alone, she has shown the champion Dane, "Special K," in 140 shows. During the long drives she often amuses herself chatting with truckers on her CB radio. I have spoken to Ms. Basquette on the telephone and her voice sounds like that of a woman of about thirty, so it's no wonder she, as she puts it, has a lot of fun with the truckers. "From the sound of my voice they all think I'm some young chick. I don't make dates with them, though. At that point, I always say, 'Oh, listen, son, I'm old enough to be your grandmother.'"

Lina Basquette was born April 19, 1907. She described her first professional appearance at the San Francisco World's Fair at the age of seven with a little chuckle in her voice, "I performed as this marvelous little child prodigy dancing on a platform with a Victor gramophone and the dog." Basquette has apparently never stopped dancing since. When I asked her if she had ever thought of retirement, she said bluntly, "If I retired I think I would disintegrate. I've never known any long periods of leisure—I'm the type who likes to do everything myself. Take the stick shift for example—I think I was the last one to go automatic. I don't think I'll ever become attuned to the push button age. I like to do everything by hand—never had a dishwasher in my house."

She moved on to dance with the Ziegfeld Follies and then to star in the Cecil B. deMille film *The Godless Girl*, which brought her, among many, a fan letter signed: Adolf Hitler! Since the name meant nothing to an American at that time, she didn't bother to have it translated and didn't save it. Later, she chanced to meet Hitler, by then all too well known, when she was taken by a friend for a weekend at his famous Bavarian retreat, the Eagle's Nest. "Hitler was no buffoon," she said in reply to my question. "He spoke English fairly well, and I spoke enough German to be cute with him. But when he didn't want to understand, he just looked blank and didn't understand." "I can assure you he was not, as some say, gay," she added. "I'm probably the only person alive who kneed him in the groin for making a pass." After that incident she left the "Eagle" in some pain in his "Nest" and got out of Germany as quickly as possible.

Retirement to What?

Basquette continued in show business into the early forties, and she managed to avoid the excesses so common to that ambience. Never entrapped by alcohol or drugs, she says maybe it was just good common sense. "I don't mind having a drink before dinner," she says, "but in a way, I've been in training for something all my life. Anything to excess, like that," she says, "bothers me. Except getting married—nine times—I never minded that."

Her theatrical career, the people she knew, and her stories of running around the world seem to lend an aura of wealth to this lady. But when I asked her, she said, "Except for a few rare periods in my life, I've never been able to sit back and just let the money roll in. I think maybe that's one of the reasons I'm as healthy as I am. When people get too much—have it too easy—they get soft."

"Now, at 78," I asked her, "what are your satisfactions in life? What are your expectations?"

"The satisfaction I get these days is to wake up in good health, be able to jump out of bed, and be able to go right on doing what I'm doing."

"Run" and "jump"—I've noticed that these same two words occur and reoccur in Basquette's chatting about herself. They not only say something about her energy level but, it seems to me, they also say a lot about her mental slant on life. She has a vigorous, optimistic attitude toward life because she's healthy and enjoys a high energy level. Or is she healthy and energetic as a *result* of her mental attitude toward life? From what I've seen, I opt for the latter.

"Of course I go to bed earlier now than when I was in show business—usually soon after the 11 o'clock news. And I'm up every day around half past four or five o'clock. I've always been able to get by on five or six hours of sleep."

"As you look toward the year 2000, what thoughts do you have?"

"I don't want to live any longer than when I can take care of myself and run around. I don't want to live a day longer than that. I'll just keep going until my time is up. I've always been a fatalist. I'm not terribly religious, but I have a great feeling of the Divinity. And I feel when your time is up, it's up.

"I don't bother with a lot of doctors and medicine and all that. And all this fear stuff that's going around—actually, I think today some of these people are making a fortune out of scaring other people. And I'm really appalled at the measures some people take to add another day or two to their lives."

As one who is alive today, thanks to some very skillful heart surgery fourteen years ago, I can't say I'm a medical nihilist, yet I do and always have subscribed to Basquette's attitude toward medicine. When I need it I'll come running, but for the rest of the time, it's hardly something to dwell on.

Finally, what about another retirement? "Well, I may retire at the end of this year, when this Great Dane is retired," replied Basquette. "Then I'll probably become a judge—or a truck driver."

BENJAMIN FRANKLIN WAS able to retire at forty-two; that is, retire from the business of making money as a printer. He then turned to science, expanded his study of electricity, tried local politics, and then, by stages, moved into the field of diplomacy. Yet, when we find him in Paris, ambassador from the revolutionary government of the colonies thirty years later, he has set up and staffed a printing press near his home. He maintained a continuing interest in everything that came to his hand.

In the early 1800s, American clipper ship captains commonly retired rich men in their late twenties or early thirties and immediately took up new careers in business and commerce. Today more and more Americans are retiring in their fifties and even forties to turn to a totally new kind of life. Businessmen move from a big city to Vermont and start farming. Couples buy an old house, work on it for a year, and soon open a new country inn with a restaurant.

Is there something to be learned from these people about what I call "retirement shock"? I think maybe yes—several things. Retirement can kill and all too often does. Yet, in the case of many men and women, retirement, at any age, has meant clearly a rebirth. There are, it seems to me, two courses open to us. If we enjoy what we are doing,

Retirement to What?

if we love what we are doing with a passion, then let's keep at it—as long as we breathe.

Mandatory retirement? That needn't stop us. What we do is no monopoly of the organization we work for. A printer can print whether in Philadelphia or Paris. A middle manager can manage at IBM or in his local town government or as a volunteer for SCORE (Service Corps of Retired Executives). Neither managing, filing, typing, designing, painting (houses or canvasses), nor counseling belongs to any single company or government department. If forced to retire, it's almost always possible to continue what you were doing in another setting. The only mistake is when the unimaginative accept the gold watch as the end. Retirement to idleness can be dangerous. Retirement to a new freedom can be exhilarating.

4

Life Expectancy

O excellent! I love long life better than figs.
—Shakespeare

Freshman year at college, I had a biology professor who wore a very unusual watch fob. Naturally, in 1937, he wore a vest, and the gold fob that graced it contained a small amount of water. In that water floated his pet amoeba, whose entire sex life consisted of dividing into two amoebas. At the end of each day my professor would remove one of the amoebas, keeping the population in his fob at one. He told us as we began our study of biology, that his pet was then twenty-six years old and that his experiment was to determine the life expectancy of an amoeba. Today that amoeba must be somewhere in its middle seventies, and, unlike my professor, it apparently has an infinite life expectancy.

The question of life expectancy has always fascinated man. Of course, the real question is "How long will *I* live?" Methuselah was said to have lived 969 years. But now we have discovered that a year, as counted then, was a lunar month, twenty-eight days, making Methuselah somewhere near eighty years old when he died—a good age but not a record even for his time. For the life span of man at that time, according to evidence now available, was probably around one hundred years—just as it is today.

Before confusion develops, we'd better define "life span" and "life expectancy." By general agreement scientists have defined life span to mean the age a species can attain naturally if its life is not cut off by disease, accident, destruction, or other interference. For example: There are English oaks casting shade today in Britain that were saplings before the occupying Romans left in the fifth century. There are somewhat more than thirty-two thousand Americans living today who were born more than one hundred years ago. The well-known redwoods make it to two thousand years and more, while the fruit fly (drosophila) lives a matter of hours. I was astounded to learn that in spite of all the changes over the past few thousand years, there is no evidence that man's life span has either lengthened or decreased measurably. All the evidence indicates that it is just beyond one hundred years.

Man's *life expectancy*, by contrast, has altered drastically over the years. Definition: the number of years an individual will still have to live if he keeps to the statistical average. During the Bronze Age in Greece, a child's life expectancy at birth was about eighteen years! Natural selection was really truckin' in those days! You had to be tough to live long enough to procreate and almost immediately shuffle off this mortal coil. Yet life span, as we defined it, was as always way up there—some did make it to one hundred.

What a lot of malarkey, you say? Who kept records in prehistory? Who indeed? The answer: bones; bones and graveyards. Back as far as one hundred thousand years ago, man made grave sites and buried all who died from a tribe or group at the same site for periods of many years. Today, scientists can ascertain age and sex from a bone or skull. Incidentally, in those days, the males lived far longer than the females. It wasn't until relatively recently that women began living noticeably longer than men.

So scientists have given us life expectancy information from prehistoric times by studying all of the skeletons buried at a single grave site. Naturally, the information is not exact, but there is sufficient agreement among different studies to guarantee fair accuracy. By Roman times your actuaries were already hard at work (annuities were not unknown even then), and life expectancies of between twenty-two and

AVERAGE LENGTH OF LIFE FROM ANCIENT TO MODERN TIMES

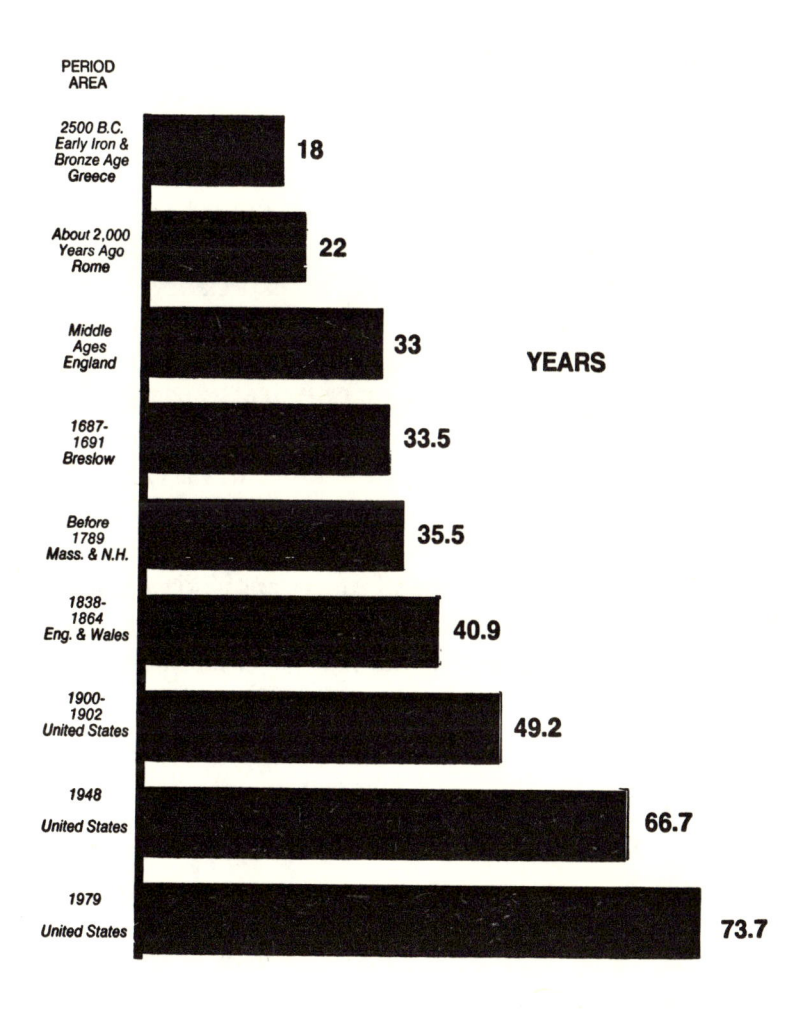

PERIOD / AREA	YEARS
2500 B.C. Early Iron & Bronze Age Greece	18
About 2,000 Years Ago Rome	22
Middle Ages England	33
1687-1691 Breslow	33.5
Before 1789 Mass. & N.H.	35.5
1838-1864 Eng. & Wales	40.9
1900-1902 United States	49.2
1948 United States	66.7
1979 United States	73.7

thirty years were projected for a Roman child at birth. And at that same time we know that, in Roman Egypt, life expectancy *at age sixty* was about fourteen years, that is, the average sixty-year-old lived to seventy-four. Look at this chart made up from a number of different sources. It gives a pretty accurate picture of human life expectancy at birth, from 2500 B.C. to the present.

Today, by the time you have reached sixty years old, the age to which you can expect to live is a lot greater than it was when you were born. So if you had made it to sixty by 1979, you then had a life expectancy of twenty more years (average) or eighty! And if you were eighty in 1979, you had a life expectancy of 8.4 years, or eighty-eight plus! Stranger and stranger, it begins to sound like *Alice in Wonderland,* but the longer you live, the longer you can expect to live.

Remember we are still talking about life expectancy, an average, not about life span. A child born in London in 1905 would undergo the risk of bombs dropped by German dirigibles in World War I, a risk not run by children living in Scotland. Children of 1905 born almost anywhere in the world were in serious danger from the great Spanish flu epidemic of 1918. In fact, my grandfather was a victim of that terrible epidemic. He died in 1918 at the age of sixty-one, when he had a theoretical life expectancy of 15.7 years, or almost to age seventy-seven. Nevertheless, the average of all Americans who were sixty-one during that epidemic did live to seventy-seven years of age. And one, his wife and my grandmother, also sixty-one, lived another thirty-four years to the age of ninety-five.

So it's the intervention of some catastrophic incident that turns life *span* into life *expectancy.* Modern medicine has worked wonders in bringing life expectancy closer to life span for all of us—but especially for the young. The thing that completely astounded me is how little life expectancy has changed over the centuries for people over fifty.

I think, like most people, I always knew that a boy or girl born in the Bronze Age or during the Middle Ages probably had a very short life ahead of him, maybe somewhere around twenty-five years—a guess that wasn't very far out. I also thought that a sixty-year-old must have been feeble with old age in those days and probably hadn't long

EXPECTATION OF LIFE PER 1,000 AMONG WHITE MALES AND WHITE FEMALES IN THE UNITED STATES FROM 1850 TO 1946 FOR THE DECENNIAL AGES OF LIFE

Sex and Calendar Period	\multicolumn{9}{c}{AGE}
	0	10	20	30	40	50	60	70	80
	\multicolumn{9}{c}{Expectation of Life, Years}
White males:									
1850	38.3	48.0	40.1	34.0	27.9	21.6	15.6	10.2	5.9
1890	42.50	48.45	40.66	34.05	27.37	20.72	14.73	9.35	5.40
1900-1902	48.23	50.59	42.19	34.88	27.74	20.76	14.35	9.03	5.10
1901-1910	49.32	50.86	42.39	34.80	27.55	20.59	14.17	8.96	5.07
1909-1911	50.23	51.32	42.71	34.87	27.43	20.39	13.98	8.83	5.09
1919-1921	56.34	54.15	45.60	37.65	29.86	22.22	15.25	9.51	5.47
1920-1929	57.85	54.65	45.84	37.51	29.35	21.65	14.75	9.17	5.26
1929-1931	59.12	54.96	46.02	37.54	29.22	21.51	14.72	9.20	5.26
1930-1939	60.62	55.86	46.77	38.06	29.57	21.71	14.86	9.29	5.30
1939-1941	62.81	57.03	47.76	38.80	30.03	21.96	15.05	9.42	5.38
1945	64.44	57.92	48.59	39.46	30.55	22.38	15.40	9.86	*
1946	65.12	58.35	48.98	39.87	30.91	22.67	15.64	10.03	*
White females:									
1850	40.5	47.2	40.2	35.4	29.8	23.5	17.0	11.3	6.4
1890	44.46	49.62	42.03	35.36	28.76	22.09	15.70	10.15	5.75
1900-1902	51.08	52.15	43.77	36.42	29.17	21.89	15.23	9.59	5.50
1901-1910	52.54	52.89	44.39	36.75	29.28	21.86	15.09	9.52	5.43
1909-1911	53.62	53.57	44.88	36.96	29.26	21.74	14.92	9.38	5.35
1919-1921	58.53	55.17	46.46	38.72	30.94	23.12	15.93	9.94	5.70
1920-1929	60.62	56.41	47.46	39.20	30.97	22.97	15.70	9.71	5.46
1929-1931	62.67	57.65	48.52	39.99	31.52	23.41	16.05	9.98	5.63
1930-1939	64.52	58.98	49.71	40.90	32.24	23.96	16.44	10.19	5.76
1939-1941	67.29	60.85	51.38	42.21	33.25	24.72	17.00	10.50	5.88
1945	69.54	62.44	52.88	43.52	34.41	25.73	17.80	11.18	*
1946	70.28	62.96	53.36	43.97	34.79	26.04	18.05	11.33	*

*Not available.

Reprinted with permission, the Ronald Press Co., New York.

to live—a guess that was wrong, very wrong! A sixty-year-old Egyptian, living at the time of Ptolemy XII (about 55 B.C.) had a life expectancy of fourteen years, to age seventy-four. Pretty close to the same figures apply to the Middle Ages. Studies made covering the seventeenth century in Europe show a sixty-year-old doing not quite as well—life expectancy of twelve years. Coming way forward to 1939, our sixty-year-old now has an expected sixteen years, to age seventy-six. So between the rules of Ptolemy XII and Roosevelt II, our sixty-year-old has gained but two years.

So it probably won't surprise you that eighty-year-olds have been doing about as well. In Ptolemy's day the eighty-year-old looked forward to about eight more years, age eighty-eight. In the Middle Ages his expectations had dropped to five years, age eighty-five. By 1939, our octogenarian had climbed back to a life expectancy of five and one-half years, say nearly eighty-six. And by 1979, he had reached an expectancy of 8.4 years, little more than in 50 B.C.!

Take a look at the chart showing life expectancies at various ages from 1850 to 1946. Particularly, look down the columns under "0" and "60."

Reading down the column under "0," we see years expected at birth rising steadily for males from thirty-eight on up to sixty-five. Then for females we see the numbers go from forty right on up to seventy without hesitation. Now look under "60" for expected years of life for males. Between 1850 and 1946, the numbers start at 15.6, rise slightly, then sag and rise again to finish at 15.64—almost no change. And for females, the figure starts at seventeen, sags and then rises slowly to 18.05.

How can one explain the tremendous change in life expectancies at birth over the past two thousand years and the virtual lack of change in expected life at sixty? I can only guess it must have been Charles Darwin's natural selection at work. The unfit, the weaklings, and, I guess, the unluckies had all been selected out after sixty years of toiling and moiling both in the days of Ptolemy and Roosevelt. And today modern medicine is succeeding in keeping the unfit and the weaklings, but not the unluckies, alive for a far greater number of

Life Expectancy

years. Happily, this medicine is also often making the unfit, fit; and the weaklings, strong.

Alas for the unluckies, heavy things fall on them and run into them, probably with greater frequency than in the past. Although I don't intend to go into causes of death in a big way, I was astonished to discover that among Americans who did die between fifteen and twenty-four years of age, three out of four died as a result of murder, accident, or suicide. I'd always thought of diseases as the major villains; but here we find that 75 percent of this group have been killing each other or themselves. So said the United Press on January 8, 1983, in an article reporting that death rates were declining for all Americans except young people. From other studies I find one more point that stands out like a sore thumb. Relative to total population, the number of accidental deaths and suicides in the United States is almost exactly double the number in Great Britain.

In case I've given the impression that modern medicine has done little toward increasing life expectancies for us "over-sixties," let me hasten to correct it. Between 55 B.C. and A.D. 1939, we found that the sixty-year-old's life expectancy had increased by only two years. That's over a period of two thousand years. Now, in only forty years (1939 to 1979, latest figures), his life expectancy has increased twice as much, that is, four years more. Instead of sixteen years, the average sixty-year-old can expect another twenty years, to age eighty. I have not separated the men from the women in these figures, so you can bear in mind that the ladies usually do a couple of years better than the average and men a little less. Incidentally, as age increases, the difference decreases. By eighty-five there is only a difference of a year and a half between the life expectancy of a man and a woman, that is, to ages ninety and a half, and ninety-two, respectively.

Anyway, enough of statistics. Instead take another look at the title of this chapter, *Life Expectancy*, a two-headed title if ever I saw one. The first meaning is the one we've been discussing, How long can we expect to live? The other, and more important one, is how *good* do we expect to live—what do we expect from life?

Here is an area in which I think both we and others constantly do ourselves a great disservice. Even our friends and physicians fall into the age-image trap here. A thirty-five-year-old announces that he has a pain in the right shoulder; it hurts when he raises his arm above a certain level. "That's terrible," say his friends and doctor, "we'll have to find out what's wrong and set it right." Then a seventy-five-year-old says the same thing. What do they tell him? "Oh, that's too bad, but what do you expect? You're not thirty-five anymore." EXPECT! I expect to be able to raise my arm over my head when I'm ninety-five. And if I can't, I expect my doctor to find out why. If there's a valid reason—some muscular problem or arthritis—okay. But let's not start with the expectation that because I'm over seventy everything should be breaking down.

Expectations have one characteristic that can either be a great help to you or do you great harm; they tend to fulfill themselves. I remember an old war story that illustrates the point nicely. A Royal Air Force (RAF) squadron commander is talking to his fighter pilots. "There are two kinds of pilots," he says, "those who go out to shoot, and those who go out to get shot at." And he went on to explain that each generally got what he expected.

Take something as simple as this: What do you expect in the way of physical comfort as you make your way through each day? For example, what about the chair you sit in more than any other—the one you choose for reading, watching television, listening to music? Is it truly comfortable? Is it a positively pleasurable sensation to ease yourself down among its cushions and lean back against a firm but soft support? Yes? Honestly? Or are you maybe mumbling to yourself, Well, it's not bad? Tell me, can you think of a chair in a friend's house that you find more comfortable than your own? I can. I was baby-sitting for my daughter's two children the other night (her husband was on a business trip) while she and my wife went to a ceramics class. Now he's got a chair—one of those that goes back while a footrest rises miraculously from nowhere. Man, that's comfort! I nearly dozed off watching a fairly good television show. Now that I'm thinking about comfort and expectations, why don't I have one; or why don't I think of buying one?

Life Expectancy

The truth? I'm not really sure. New England Puritan background? It's decadent—effete? Expensive! That's it—though I don't even know what such a chair would cost. Whatever it costs, it's too much to spend just to be comfortable; my present wooden armchair was good enough for the early colonists, it's good enough for me. That's the truth—right off the top of my head. And, now that I think of it, what's the matter with me? Answer: My expectations are too low. I just don't expect much in the comfort department and so, as the night follows the day, I don't get much.

This is, I think, the more important aspect of life expectancy. This is not twenty-three or fifteen years from now. This is today, tomorrow, the next day. This is NOW. And here's an aspect of my life where I'm *underexpecting*. And if there's one such area, you can be sure there are others. What about your shoes? Are your feet comfortable when you take long walks? when you work in the garden? or when you are just slouching around the house? What about your car? Would you feel more comfortable with a good back cushion? And how's that pallet you sleep on? Webster defines a pallet as "a straw bed or mattress, often connoting a poor or inferior bed." Do you sleep in dreamless luxury on a couch fit for emperors?—or on a pallet? Whatever it is, you can be sure that it's the result of your expectations—or lack thereof. Remember physical comfort is very important to good living. It affects your outlook on the whole day, your disposition—sunny or cloudy. How can anyone whose feet hurt from the wrong shoes, or whose back aches from a poorly designed chair, meet the events and people of the day with a smile and expectations of good things? Most of us who are now over sixty inherited, as a general rule, the idea that if it tastes bad it must be good for you; that if it feels good, there must be something morally wrong about it; that if it's really comfortable, it's best described as sinfully comfortable.

If you try to trace the false syllogism that if it's comfortable it must be wrong, I think you'll find that it descends from situations in which discomfort was inevitable and comfort could not be expected. Whether you came to America on a slave ship or the *Mayflower*, it was probably more uncomfortable than anything any of us has experienced today; and there was no choice but to bear it. I certainly can't conceive of what it must have been like to go to Utah in a covered wagon, but to complain about it all the way from New York to Salt Lake City was certainly sinful.

So let's agree that comfort is good for you. In situations in which you can't have it, the drill is: Grin and bear it. But when comfort is available, for heaven's sake get comfortable.

Take a look at your social life and your expectations there. Is a variety of companionship what you want? And, if you want it, are you getting it? The father-in-law of one of my sons will be getting his B.A. this spring. A retiree from the air force, he's been taking courses, somewhat haphazardly, for a number of years; and now, he finds, he has the required credits and is about to don a cap and gown. He's in his sixties and has no particular need for the degree. His real reason for taking the courses over the years was mainly social—he wanted to meet regularly with different people with different interests and of different ages. And he found adult education courses a good way to do it.

Ordinarily, in the course of a working life, one has contact with a lot of different people every day. Then, suddenly, on retirement, we find our circle of acquaintances shrinking down to a few (and not all so precious). It's not necessary. With few exceptions, if we look, we'll find some kind of senior citizen center within a few miles of where we live. And, if it's a well-run one, the variety of people and activities you'll find there is surprising. But if you've tried your local center and found it to be nothing but a group of old fogies, well there are plenty of other ways to expand your circle of contacts. In fact, it's a mistake to count on a senior citizen group as your only source of social contacts for the simple reason that it limits you to older people. The variety of views that a cross section of people of all ages exposes you to continually challenges your mind, keeping it healthy and flexible.

There are literally dozens of special interest groups that will welcome your participation. They are to be found under such headings as athletic, political, literary, foreign language, bird watchers, horicultural, and many others. Then there are the volunteer organizations, more rich sources of human contact that can add variety and interest to your life. You might choose to work once or twice a week in a hospital; to visit occasionally with at-home shut-ins who suffer from lack of human contact; or to join SCORE, a group of retired executives who help young businessmen solve the same problems they mastered years ago. Try 'em, one after the other, until you find the activity that gives you the variety of human contacts you're looking for.

Here's another area in which you may or may not have expectations; your intellectual life. No, I'm not talking about the ideas of Hegel or Kant, or of Boolean algebra or oriental philosophy. I'm referring to those things that may please your mind, your eye, your ear. It's quite possible that there may be art forms you have never explored that could touch you deeply and could quickly become an important part of your life interests. Take the case of the artist Harry Lieberman, who died not long ago at the age of 106. He spent most of his life in the wholesale confectioner business. Then, in his seventies, he retired, soon became bored with that, and decided to try his hand at sketching at the Great Neck Golden Age Club on Long Island. His efforts blossomed into a new career in watercolors and oil painting, and his works have since been shown at the Hirshhorn Museum, Washington, D.C., and museums in Houston, Seattle, Los Angeles, and Rotterdam, Holland.

Are you a good writer; a good reader? I'm not absolutely sure which calls for the greater skill. I know without question that for me the written word has transported me further throughout the world and universe, and further into the minds and souls of man, than any firsthand physical experience could have done. Of course, there are certain experiences that have to be lived to be known. However, the vast majority of experience is not available to us firsthand for reasons of time and space; for example, what life was like in the Middle Ages, or what is the appearance of Arcturus close up. But there is a marvelous time-space machine always available to you, and it's closer than you think. Your local library! And don't say "Ohhhh" on a descending note. If you don't agree, maybe you're not a reader.

LIFE BEGINS AT SIXTY

There are many such people. It's probably something tricky to do with the eye or nerve route to the brain or synapses or something. But lack of a desire to read need hardly cripple your intellectual life. You have the theater, movies, television, museums—sources of endless material that can bring surprise and pleasure to all your senses. Yet, always, the key to your enjoyment of them remains: your expectations. This applies, I firmly believe, to every part of your life—your sex life, your enjoyment of eating and drinking, how well you sleep at night, the respect you receive from others, and even your spiritual life.

In no way am I attempting to convince you that if you just want something enough, you'll get it. This is the real world we're talking about. And I'm perfectly aware that people often entertain what are known as false expectations. What we're talking about here are realistic ones in the real world you recognize you live in. Anything is possible; fewer things are probable; don't diminish them further through low expectations.

5

To What Purpose?

The aim, if reached or not, makes great the life.
—Browning

When my eyes open in the morning, after taking a look at my sleeping wife's face on the pillow next to me, I contemplate the day and what I'm going to do with it. Over the centuries people have opened their eyes to purposes of many varieties and magnitude—to the purpose of landing an army on the beaches of Normandy; to the purpose of at last breaking eighty on the local golf course; to the purpose of transplanting a new heart where an old one was failing; to the purpose of pursuading that lovely girl to say *yes* before the day is done; to the purpose of closing that long hanging real estate deal.

All of these provide good reasons for meeting the day with vigor and expectation. Conversely, a day with no goal, not even the goal of creative loafing, is condemned to be a day of aging and nothing else.

A word about creative loafing and other such less than noble goals: Whether noble or ignoble, a goal—any goal—lends vigor, direction, and vitality to the person pursuing it. Apparently, evil goals are just as good for the health of whoever pursues them as admirable goals. More evil goals can scarcely be imagined than those of Adolf Hitler, yet until, in the last years of World War II, he witnessed the crushing of his violent hopes, he pursued them with the greatest vitality.

LIFE BEGINS AT SIXTY

Revenge is another perhaps ignoble goal that seems to lend superhuman strength and endurance to those obsessed by it. Such people will go to the ends of the earth untouched by disease and hardships, whatever is placed in their way, until they achieve their goal. There are countless instances of men who have endured years in prison, patiently awaiting the day when they would be set free to wreak their vengeance.

Like greatness, goals are sometimes achieved by us and sometimes thrust upon us. When a good goal is "thrust upon us," we can accept it with thanks. But during the years after sixty, it is less likely that goals will be handed to us. Then, time forces us to take our fate into our own hands.

I think you can probably divide goals roughly into three categories: long term, intermediate, and short term. Dorothy Fuldheim, that remarkable television commentator from Cleveland, and I didn't discuss goals as such, but as a result of my interviews with her, I'd say her goals fell into those categories. Her most important long-term goal was to "leave enough for my granddaughter," who, you may remember, could not take care of herself. Not long ago, she had an intermediate goal of getting a raise and a new contract as she turned ninety. She got both and made international news doing so. But Fuldheim also set day-to-day short-term goals, preparing what she would say three times a day on WSEW-TV in Cleveland. In her case the three kinds of goals are closely interrelated and, in a practical sense, sometimes almost indistinguishable; and this is usually so for anyone pursuing a career that has filled most of their life.

But most of us retire at some point. Then, it is up to us to manufacture or discover our own goals—or live without them. But a life without goals is, by definition, no life at all. A person with no *raison d'être* will not être very long. And since the point of this book is to find ways of living longer and with more fun, we'd better find out how to discover or make goals for ourselves.

How have others done it? Harry Lieberman, the confectioner we mentioned in the last chapter, who retired and became an artist, got the idea for that vital change in his life when his eye was caught by an

To What Purpose?

announcement of sketching classes, an activity in which he thought he might have some ability. When he tried it, he found he had uncovered the possibility of expressing himself in a medium he had never tried before. It turned out to be the beginning of a twenty-six-year career. I can't prove that Lieberman lived happily and productively to the age of 106 because he set for himself the goal of becoming a recognized artist—because when he was almost eighty he found a new reason for getting up in the morning. But I know what I think. It's a little like the joke about the hundred-year-old man who said, "If I'd known I was going to live this long, I'd have taken better care of myself." If you live to be 106, you may wind up saying, "If I'd known I was going to live this long, I'd have found something more interesting to do."

Harry Lieberman discovered within himself an unusual talent, and his work ended up in museums. But we don't need fame and recognition from achieving our goals. Take a look at Roy Hutchings, born in England, an RAF pilot during World War II, followed by a full career as a mechanical engineer. He retired in 1977 because heavy travel was affecting his health. "I was frequently scheduled for Monday morning meetings as far away as North Africa, England, or California," Hutchings explains. He was based in Stamford, Connecticut, and that meant "losing weekend after weekend. I found it particularly draining in the winter." A careful check of finances showed retirement to be feasible and so Roy and his wife, Joyce, took the plunge. "It's not a bridge you burn down," he said. "You can always go back over it. In fact I have several friends who retired, tried it out for a year, didn't like it, and went back to work." One might argue that not everyone could return to the job they retired from and that many would find it difficult to return to the job market in their sixties. But we're talking about goals, and Hutchings had achieved his first goal: He was no longer tied to regular employment.

There was a short period Hutchings said, when he didn't know what to do—a slowing down into a new tempo. After all, he hadn't retired for a positive purpose but rather to get away from something. What followed was probably fairly common to most retirees, a slow development of a number of different purposes in his life. None of these goals was earth shattering; on the other hand, without them his life might well have deteriorated. Hutchings had a daughter living in California whom he had not really seen for many years, and so his first goal became the planning of an extended visit "to see her and get acquainted again. That, we decided would be our first major project." For the very affluent, the project might have been ultra simple. For most of us living on retirement income, however, it deserves to be called a major project.

Achieve it they did, however, as Hutchings and his wife flew to California, rented a car, and got to know their daughter again. They also did a little reconnoitering, fell in love with California, and almost chose, as a further goal, moving to the West Coast. "Almost" because they found that a house where they wanted it in California would cost three times what they could hope to get for their house in Connecticut.

"There was a little bit of a slowdown after that," Hutchings said, "but I finally began to look around for other things." Going on in Hutching's mind was the process of achieving a goal. "I've always been interested in wood. In fact, I still have a piece of wood I carved when I was fourteen years old. It's an oak sphere. Looking at it, I realized how much I liked making things of wood, and I began to look around to see what was needed."

Although he had a few woodworking tools, Hutchings did not have any of the machinery that he felt was necessary for really accomplishing something. But at a local high school, he found evening adult education courses in woodworking. "Attending these classes allowed me to use the tools, and since the class instructor was a sculptor, he had a wide selection of them. This was important because I was interested in sculpting things out of wood."

Directly after the war, Hutching's work took him to Kenya, where he immediately fell in love with the variety of animal life. This interest has stuck with him, and now, more than thirty years later, his sculpture has developed around the theme of wild animals. In his living room stands an African elephant about one foot tall, sculptured

To What Purpose?

out of rich, brown California sugar pine. The tusks are of contrasting white cedar, and the toenails (white) are carved from a steak bone. For eyes, which are relatively small, Hutchings used black beads. Trunk partly raised, the animal is startlingly lifelike—an inhabitant of the African plains, caught in the midst of life, and frozen in time like a flash of memory.

Now, you will expect me to tell you that Hutchings's works have been collected by this museum and that, and that they sell for X number of dollars. Not the case here. Roy Hutchings's animals and birds serve to fulfill something creative in him, and that's all he wants from them. "I decided on no competitions because my aim was for this to be something I could relax with. I couldn't see getting into competition or going into selling. That would turn it into a commercial type of operation, and that's what I wanted to stay away from. So, no exhibits—I'd only make carvings for gifts." Hutchings has friends throughout the world, and that is where his works have found their home. The only exception is his senior citizens center. He did get talked into making things for display and to sell there. Some of the money goes to the center and some to the purchase of tools and materials for Hutchings's work.

Here are a few of his favorite things: "being at the bench with my favorite tools, lots of wood, creating things that result in something pleasing to the eye, feeling the enjoyment of having made it, and putting myself into the design and accomplishment of the piece—feeling the pleasure of giving it away and seeing the receiver pleased at getting something handmade, that you can't buy or go out and duplicate, seeing that what I create is giving some child somewhere a lot of pleasure."

Roy Hutchings is seventy-one now, and I wouldn't be at all surprised to see him at his bench twenty years from now, turning out new and different works of art.

IF HE DOES that, he will still be a year younger than Ruby Hemenway was when she wrote her first weekly column for the *Greenfield Recorder*. For it is in Turners Falls, Massachusetts, where the Connecticut River comes roaring down from Vermont, that Ruby Hemenway, at ninety-two, composed her first newspaper column in 1976. A few of her reminiscences had appeared earlier in a historical column; and when that columnist, far younger than Ruby, approached his retirement, he suggested that she take over the column. With characteristic verve she took on the job and completed eight years of the weekly stint in January 1984, when she reached one hundred.

I was intensely curious as to what kind of a person this could be who would embark on a new career at ninety-two years of age. What I found was a very likable lady—a very normal human being.

I asked her to think back to her eightieth birthday and the goals that seemed important to her then. Had she accomplished them? "Yes, I think I have," she said. "The main things I thought important were enjoying life, enjoying the friends around me—and the world around me. The writing helped a great deal when I got to the point that I couldn't be too active." When I followed up by asking about secondary goals in her life, she replied, "To stay healthy so that I can enjoy life as long as I live." There appeared a key word, for the fourth time: "enjoy." I suspect that the United States is the only country in the world whose founding document, the Declaration of Independence, gives "the pursuit of happiness" as one of its three basic reasons for existence. And if we listen to how all the people I've been talking to describe their years after sixty, that pursuit of happiness rings a common chord. It is a goal they all share; a goal that is quite right and proper.

I asked Miss Hemenway what her first thoughts were when she awakened every morning. "Well, I lie in bed awhile," she said, "and plan the day's work. Rather sketchily, but that's how I start. And that's where my weekly column comes in; it gives me a definite thing to be interested in, to work for, and to accomplish. It's also quite important in my life because it makes a point of contact with people." I asked her if there were other activities in her life more important than the column. Her answer was very much that of the career person. "My family and my relations are *as* important to me," with the accent on

To What Purpose?

the word "as." The weekly goal of turning out her newspaper column ranked as high as anything else in Ruby Hemenway's life.

By January 1984 Miss Hemenway had completed more than four hundred columns for the *Greenfield Recorder* when vision problems overtook her. One of the questions I had asked her was "Right now, what is your most important goal in life?" Her reply, "To get so I can see again." Her sight had been failing for some time because of cataracts, and she was finally forced to give up writing the columns. With characteristic verve, she opted for operations on both eyes and underwent the first in January; and a cataract was removed from the other eye in May. When I talked to her in June 1984, she told me, in her usual vigorous tones, "I've got to wait a month before they'll be testing my eyes for new lenses. The doctor said that he hoped then that I would be able to see as well as when I was fifty years old."

During all this conversation I was feeling a little nervous. It's not like interviewing a movie star or a politician. They're fair game and one does not worry unduly about bruising their feelings. But Ruby Hemenway is a sensitive, normal human being, who knows she's in the spotlight only because she has lived longer than most of us can hope for. So I naturally feared that my probing might make her uneasy or even angry if she felt that I was putting her under a microscope like some sort of a freak. Not at all. She put *me* at my ease, and she was delighted at my questions. "It was fun to answer something different than the same questions I've been asked so many times."

"So you're not writing your column now, of course," I assumed. Wrong! "Well, I've just written three, and I think there'll be one published today. One was published a while ago, and I'm going to try to do more." I asked her if she dictated the pieces. "You don't write them yourself now, do you?"

"Yes," was the firm reply. "It isn't very good, but they seem to be able to read it. I'd rather do it myself; I can do better than I do with dictation."

I asked her if I might call her in late July and find out how the operations worked out and how she was feeling then. "Why that would be very kind of you," she replied. What a beautiful response to what had to be regarded as a self-serving question from me. I was not being kind to her, though I was surely sincere when I wished her the best of luck.

PEOPLE TEND TO keep a great assortment of odds and ends in their basements, mostly items in limbo that the owners can't quite bring themselves to throw out. But Mary Boose keeps more than five thousand living things in her basement—things that give purpose to her life at the youthful age of seventy.

She grows African violets—more than three hundred varieties. And they all thrive under the dozens of fluorescent "grow lights" she has installed over the benches on which rest her flats of flowers, some pink, some white, some blue or lavender. I said that purpose was sometimes thrust upon us and sometimes achieved by us. In Mary's case I suspect it was a combination. Some twenty-five years ago, she chanced to see two African violet plants in a friend's house, and her enthrallment dates from that day.

Boose's involvement with African violets is not only a hobby but also a thriving business that keeps her busy more than five hours a day filling orders for plants from the farthest reaches of North America. It has also been a therapy that played an important part in her recovery from a recent heart attack.

For weeks after the attack her beloved basement garden was out of bounds because of the stairs. Then finally a physical therapist started making regular visits and helped her down. There were all her plants and there, too, were all the ribbons and trophies her plants had won for her. When her therapist was unable to visit her for several weeks, the call of her subterranean gardens proved too great, and she took to making the trip by herself.

When the therapist finally resumed his calls, it was apparent that her violets had not gone uncared for, and she admitted she had been making unauthorized trips down and up the cellar stairs. After examining her, the therapist had to confess that he could have done

To What Purpose?

nothing better for her than her beloved African violets had done. Purpose is what powers our lives. Mary Boose, at seventy, descends to take care of her plants. Ruby Hemenway at a hundred and one rises each morning to write her next column for the *Greenfield Recorder*.

NOW I WANT you to meet a man some thirteen years younger than Ruby Hemenway but, like her, still active in that he is to be found running his small grocery store seven days a week. The store is one that Jimmy Soter opened in 1924, twenty-seven years after he was born in Albania and seven years after he came to America. Jimmy never spent a day in school and for many years after coming to America was unable to read or write. The fact that he could not read meant that Jimmy's picture of life and the world was limited primarily to what he actually experienced.

His first job after he arrived was as a shoemaker, at which he earned $6.50 a week. A bed cost one dollar a week. Five dollars paid for all the food he needed. During his first six months in the United States he saved twelve dollars. Several years later, he sold his first food store for eighteen hundred dollars. That's how he learned arithmetic. Not too many years later, he was the owner of two grocery stores and a two-family house that provided substantial income, all in addition to his own house. This helped him put three children through college, one of whom is now a stockbroker in California, one an accountant, and the other runs the store. How much better would he have done with an M.B.A. from Harvard Business School?

I first met Jimmy behind the counter of his little store, where he has been presiding the last sixty years. "I'll take this *Times*, a loaf of bread and, uh, do you have clam chowder—Snow's my wife said?" The little store was jammed to the rafters, and every available space was taken with groceries, newspapers, magazines, and all the good old candies; Baby Ruth, Fifth Avenue, Hershey, and so on. The uneven floors, worn counters, "sit down" telephone booth in one corner, all contributed to the feeling of a grocery-candy store of the twenties.

"Sure we havea Snows. Whatever you wanta, we havea, you know that." The little man behind the counter smiled and fetched the soup.

LIFE BEGINS AT SIXTY

He had the accent of those foreign born who progress just so far with English and then settle for a hybrid language understandable to others yet retaining the lilt and cadence of their own. "Now letsa see." He took a brown paper bag and started writing the price of each item with a two-inch pencil stub. Like those two-day beards you see on some men that never grow and are never shaven, Jimmy Soter's pencil was eternally two inches long. And Jimmy was eternally cheerful.

Lest you think him a drudge, these days Jimmy works only from five to nine in the evening, though he is in charge seven days a week. During the day he likes to be outdoors, he says, but in the evenings he likes to chat with old customers, kiss the girls when he can, and collect a few bananas, apples, or other fruit, which are the only compensation he takes from the store now. As I paid my bill, I felt my hair blown gently by an old ceiling fan, the kind they are trying to revive today—though the new ones may not outlast Jimmy's. "We put it up in 1925," he said. "We oil it every year and it keeps working. It's never been taken down."

What does Jimmy do when he's not in the store? Jimmy had invited me to visit him at his home, and as I drove up one morning about ten, I found him working in his vegetable garden. Short, wiry, burnt brown by hours in the sun, Jimmy looked like an Indian as he came out of his corn patch. The garden was about sixty feet long by thirty feet, and I saw tomatoes, peppers, ochra, beans, eggplant, cucumbers, and more, in addition to the stand of corn. A good piece of work for an eighty-seven-year-old. But he had further outdoor interests, I learned. The town had cut down two dead trees in front of his house and, at his request, left all the main branches on his property. In addition there was a dying cherry tree. All of this wood was destined for his fireplace, and Jimmy worked in a leisurely but steady fashion with ax, wedges, and saw to enlarge his already substantial woodpile.

That's a pretty big wedge, I said looking at his sledge hammer and wedge. "Twelve pounds," he said proudly. "I gotta two—so if one gets stuck." I knew what he meant, having lost more than one wedge in a stubborn piece of oak.

We walked along looking at the vigorous plants in his weed-free

To What Purpose?

garden. "Can you guess what'sa this?" he asked, indicating a plant that stood alone, maybe two feet tall.

"Gardenia," I tried.

"Orange tree," he said. I take seeds from an orange and plant." It had been an experiment. The year before, he told me, he had tried celery for the first time. "I put on manure samea everything else," he explained. "And it dried up. Leaves turn yellow, turn to powder and fall off. Now look," he pointed proudly to this year's plants. "No manure." Indeed the celery was thriving.

We went inside to talk. His house was a small Cape Cod model: two storied, two bedrooms, nice large kitchen. He had built the house five years earlier on a plot behind the large Victorian house where he had lived until his wife's death. We sat at the kitchen table, and he heated water in a pan to make instant coffee for both of us. I spooned coffee into my cup, and when the water boiled, he brought the pan to the table. He held it in one hand and I have to admit I worried about a spill as he held it over my cup, but his hand was as steady as a robot's arm as he twisted the pan and filled my cup neatly to the brim.

When I had pulled my chair back to sit down, I'd noticed a burn about eight inches long on the floor. "What happened?" I asked with rude curiosity.

"Tear gas," he said, smiling.

"What?"

"Two years ago," he started, preparing to tell a story he obviously enjoyed, "I rent a room upstairs to a girl." And he went on to tell me that she had brought a man and, later, another man to stay there. Apparently, this didn't bother Jimmy. However, one of the men held up a jewelry store, killing a clerk in the process. Jimmy didn't know this when one night he received a call from the chief of police, telling him to get down to his store right away. He went and was then told of a coming police raid on his house. Twelve cops surrounded the house, shouted an ultimatum, and, then, stormed the place with tear gas, guns, and so on. "Broke all the windows," said Jimmy. "And when they get upstairs, nobody there." It turned out that, later, they caught the man but never, after two years, found a trace of the girl.

LIFE BEGINS AT SIXTY

The police reassured Jimmy that insurance would cover the damage, but as it turned out, a hitch somewhere prevented that. Jimmy laughed as if at something that didn't concern him. "So, cost me two thousand dollar." I noticed he always had a way of laughing at money problems as if they were somehow unreal. A year or so ago, he sent eleven thousand dollars to his broker son in California to invest in oil. Now he showed me a statement from the brokerage house showing assets of sixty-five hundred dollars. "I lose five thousand dollar," he told me, laughing uproariously. "Five thousand dollar!" To him it was hilarious. The reality of money to Jimmy was $6.50 coming in a week and $6.00 going out. That's making money.

THIS CHAPTER IS supposed to be about goals. A funny thing about goals is that it doesn't seem to matter much what they are—as long as you have them. Columbus's goal was not to sail *around* the world or to prove that it is a globe. Let's face it, his goal was to make money trading with the Indies.

I doubt if Jimmy Soter ever verbalized his goals—at least not as such. I'm not going to lay them out in front of you either. But it wouldn't be a bad idea to ponder what his were—as an emigrant from Albania, as a shoemaker at $6.50 a week, as a store owner, as a father of three, as a gardener today, and as a socializing host in the Soter grocery store every day from five to nine.

To what purpose does the sun rise? Man has wrestled with the grand question over the millenia. Don't search for answers in the vast black depths among the galaxies. The sun rises to warm the bones of the old man on the park bench, to brown the skin of a girl on a beach.

6

Doing Good

Tis only noble to be good.
Kind hearts are more than coronets.
—Tennyson

The sudden ring of the telephone broke the concentration of the man reading deep in an easy chair in the comfortably furnished living room. He put down the book and crossed to pick up the telephone. "Good morning," he said in his usual cheerful voice.

"Russ?"

"This is Russell Cumming."

"Russ," the other voice hurried on, "you going to watch the Super Bowl today?"

"Oh, hello, Mark." Cumming paused a moment. He was not planning to watch the game. At the same time, he knew perfectly well that Mark was angling for an invitation. "Yeah, I thought I might take a look at it."

And so they arranged that Mark, to whom a TV set was not available, would drop over around two o'clock and watch the game with Russell.

An unremarkable conversation, you might say, and yet there was one thing about it somewhat unusual. Russell Cumming is seventy-two years old. Mark is twelve years old.

In the organization to which they both belong, Mark is known as a "little brother"; and Russell Cumming is known as his "big brother." They are not related. In fact, six months earlier they had never even met.

What do Russell and Mark have to do with the subject of this book—living a rich and rewarding life in that third period, sixty to ninety-plus? the period I've called LIVING? Answer: everything. Cumming is practicing a life principle sometimes known as "doing good." What a mundane phrase to describe the kind of exciting investment with almost the "highest yield" one can make. I've used a financial term to underline the fact that the return on the investment of doing good is quite as real as money in the bank.

It's a strange fact that the concept of doing good has many negative connotations. The phrase "do-gooders" is not usually meant as a compliment. I somehow doubt that my title for this chapter really motivates you to rush right out and look for someone who needs help.

Yet most of us are familiar with that impulse to do something for someone else whether it's sending a small check for that poor orphan in India, or giving that hopeless-looking "bag woman" in a large city five dollars for one really good hot meal. And those impulses can be pretty strong sometimes. Yet most of us (not all) usually manage to overcome the impulse. There are plenty of good reasons. "The fund-raisers probably get most of the money anyway. She'll probably spend it on a pint of gin. India! There's so much graft there the help probably wouldn't get near the poor kid in the picture." Sadly, all too often true.

But what about that impulse to help another human being? It originated in your heart. It expressed your membership in the human race. It is not good for your feelings about yourself to continually stifle such impulses. Conversely, it will contribute to your health and to a long, rich life to act on the impulse at times. When you do something good for another in some strange, mysterious way—spiritual perhaps—the act places you in touch with all the other beings who have yielded to that impulse, and you draw an immeasurable strength from the contact. So let's rescue the phrase "doing good" from its unfortu-

Doing Good

nate shadow and come right out and admit that when you give, you get.

When I talked to that "big brother," Russell Cumming, I asked him when that impulse to do something for a child in a broken family hit him. I don't think he was quite sure himself. Well, he said, his wife had died some years earlier; he was lonely, and he was looking around for some way to fill the empty hours. As head of the local National Exchange Club, he was in charge of finding speakers, and one of those he found was the director of the local Big Brothers and Sisters of America organization. And it was while listening to the speaker describe how the group helped children with only one parent that Cumming was hit by that impulse. And he didn't fight it. Now, several years later, Cummings is working with his second little brother, Mark; and he says the experience has enriched his life probably as much as any single action he has ever taken. I asked Cumming if there had been any great moment when he felt a reward for his actions.

"Maybe there was," he said. Last year, Cumming was named "Man of the Year" by Big Brothers of America. There was a ceremony for presenting the awards at which Cumming and his partner, Mark, were present. "It wasn't getting the award that was so important," he said. "No, that wasn't it. My reward came later when Mark looked up at me and said, "We did it together. We did it together, didn't we, Russ."

"I'll tell you," said Cumming, "at that moment, there was something really big caught in my throat."

Being a big brother or sister may sound demanding, and in one way, it is. Being in loco parentis for a young boy or girl is no small responsibility. On the other hand it calls for only fours a week (usually Saturdays in Cumming's case), no great organization, and the spending of money on the youngsters is discouraged. The organization structures the whole operation and relationship to place the least burden on the participants. Matching the older and younger individual is done with the greatest care. Obviously, similar interests and background are important. Cumming heard nothing for six months after making his first application. Finally, he called. Maybe I'm too old he wondered. Not at all was the answer, it's just a matter of finding the right boy for you. Cumming liked hiking, the outdoors, backpacking, and mountain climbing. He liked good music and the theater, but he was not especially interested in organized sports. Twice the organization has found boys that were right for him. The second boy, Mark had actually said, "I don't want a father. What I want is a *grandfather*." It turned out, not too surprisingly, that both of Mark's grandfathers were dead, and he felt the loss of that relationship keenly enough to be able to articulate it.

Cumming told me about one of the high points in the time spent with his first little brother, Peter. The relationship of old and young usually begins when the child is around eleven years old and terminates at the boy's or girl's sixteenth birthday. When Peter became sixteen, there was a break in the school year and Cumming asked Peter if he would like to spend a day in New York. I'll tell you the story as Cumming told it to me.

"We planned the day. Before I tell you about it, I want to specify that I cleared everything we were going to do with the boy's mother. For example, I knew he had never seen a live stage production, but I was sure surprised at what he picked. Maybe it was from television commercials, but what Peter wanted to see was *Evita*.

"So we set off at noon. I left my car at the railroad station, and right there came my first surprise. Peter had never ridden on a train in his life! Every detail was a new experience for him—the acceleration as we pulled out of the station, the friendly chat we had with the conductor, the lack of a visible engine pulling the train, and the view of the countryside from the window. But I believe the most eye-opening experiences were for me. I found myself seeing everything through Peter's eyes and, dammit, I felt sixteen not seventy as we went through that day.

"As soon as we got into the city we walked to Times Square. There's a place there where you can buy 'same day' theater tickets for half

Doing Good

price. Luckily *Evita* had had a long run and there were matinee seats, and for just eleven dollars each. On the way to the theater, we passed a teenager hustling the public with three-card monte—you know that card game where the 'sucker' tries to follow the ace of spades while the operator shuffles the three cards around face down? Peter wanted to watch. A man and a girl were also watching, and the girl urged the man to try it. To Peter's astonishment, and mine, the man put down a bet of forty dollars. It was gone in seconds. 'Did you see that?' Peter said. He could hardly believe what he had just seen, and I've got to admit my mouth was open, too. Before we knew it, the hustler had picked up his cards and vanished down the street. A policeman was approaching.

"The whole day went that way, with me seeing everything through young eyes, with me feeling younger and younger as events passed. We saw *Evita* from front row seats, Peter's idea, and I realized more acutely than ever that those were real people up there making us laugh and cry and raising our hearts with their songs. It was Peter who noticed which actors were sweating. And it was I who realized that young eyes miss very little—I noticed details I hadn't seen for years—and for those moments I had young eyes. It hit me for just a minute there that I was supposed to be doing this kid a favor, but now I couldn't say who got the most out of it.

"That was the afternoon. Then we had dinner before going on to Radio City Music Hall for the live stage show and then the movie. It was after midnight by the time we finally got back to my car at the station. And I'll tell you one thing, Peter was tired; yeah, he was about on his knees when I delivered him to his house. But one thing I was sure of: I'd given him a good day."

Notice it wasn't Russell Cumming who was tired. He was flying high—on the best kind of "restricted substance" in the world: doing good.

LET ME TELL you about a small thing I've started doing recently that is giving me a feeling of contributing to the plus side of the human condition. I had been corresponding, maybe three or four letters a year, with a friend of my father. My father died years ago, but this man, now approaching ninety, was a close friend, and our families had shared a great deal. Last Christmas, his annual card was written by his wife who told us that the Colonel, his rank on retirement from the air force, had lost his sight last year. He had been using a typewriter with double-sized type, but now, his ability to correspond was lost entirely. And the Colonel had always carried on a voluminous correspondence with people his age and down to my generation and even to the generation following mine. Many of his correspondents were well known and in positions of power and influence (for example, the president of one of the major networks); and one of the things he did was to act as a kind of clearinghouse among the lot of us. He sent copies of our letters on to others who might be interested—or should be as he saw it. Thinking about it, I realized what a terrible loss it would be to this man no longer to have this correspondence with those lively and creative minds he was used to exchanging ideas with.

But it occurred to me, correspondence need not always be written. As an editor with my old company I had often talked to the sales force through the medium of cassette tapes. I bought some C-60 (one-hour) tapes and, after some clumsy experimenting, made the first message, about forty minutes. The main problem was how to eliminate those long silences while I do what passes for thinking. My old tape recorder is not easy to stop and restart. Staring out the window and scratching one's head don't show in a written letter, but they are something less than suspenseful on a sound tape. The answer, I found, was to buy a little plug-in microphone with an "on-off" switch; an effective way of hiding my periods of creative sterility. So, off went the first effort. Nearly a month went by with no reply. Maybe my experiment was a flop; maybe my message had been so boring that a reply was impossible; or maybe it just wasn't a medium that appealed to the Colonel. Then one day, a cassette mailer appeared with the mail. It had been misaddressed, which explained the delay. And the half hour of talk was fascinating. It was full of acute and interesting observations about the world today. The Colonel told me that since losing his sight, he had become an avid radio fan, listening particularly to "talk" shows and other programs that told him what was going on in the world.

He told me with words how much he appreciated my making the tape and starting what would become a now-and-then sound letter between us. But the tone of his voice on the tape was all the thanks I could ever want for having made the small, slightly inventive, effort to keep our correspondence going. I haven't suggested it to him yet, but my real hope is that the Colonel will expand his horizons and initiate recorded correspondence with his many other friends. Fortunately, his lovely wife is in good health and is able to handle the tapes and the mailings for him.

There it is: a small effort by one human being to brighten the life of another a little bit. I can tell you from firsthand experience, it works both ways.

THERE WERE MAYBE fifty people in the room, among them people of substance in the town and the representatives of several large corporations. They were attending a reception and cocktail party in support of the Literacy Volunteers of America, a remarkable organization that was founded by Ruth Colvin in 1968 and that now teaches reading and writing, in thirty-seven states, to adult Americans who lack those skills. The main speaker was introduced; a black woman who was a housekeeper and who three years before could not read street signs or write her own name. Her volunteer teacher, Mrs. Lillian Kittner, seventy-seven years old, introduced Lola Dennis, her fifty-year-old student.

Mrs. Dennis began to explain, in her soft, southern accent, why she had never learned reading or writing. When she was six or seven and living on her parents' farm, it had been her job to take care of the younger children. A few years later, her father died, and she went to work for $7 a week in town. This was less than forty years ago. Her story caught the attention of her audience, and the memory of it brought tears to her own eyes.

Mrs. Dennis had the vision and ambition in her late forties to make herself literate. And Lillian Kittner, at seventy-seven, had the ability and the desire to help another human being. Of course, Mrs. Kittner was "doing good," but she was, possibly unknowingly, doing great good for herself at the same time.

"Mrs. Kittner," I asked, "how did you come to get involved with the Literacy Volunteers of America?"

"I had heard of the organization in town. The library had started it. I was retired and had been doing some one-to-one work with preschool children, but I guess I was looking for something more meaningful. I started with 'English as a second language' for new Americans. I'd been working with Chinese, Vietnamese—people like that. But I came to feel that my priority was with Americans, those who had somehow slipped through our educational system. And that's how I wound up working with two black Americans, Lola Dennis and Hubert Newton, who is seventy-one now. He has vowed to himself he's going to learn to read and write before he dies. We've been working for four years. That may seem long, but he had only one year of schooling."

"Well, who found who?" I asked. "How did you get together?"

"A few years ago, the local newspaper ran a full-page story about Literacy Volunteers; and it carried pictures of me and some of the others. Lola knew she wanted to read and she told me when she saw my picture she knew right then that I was the right teacher. And so we met and we began. Lately, my husband has been very sick, and I told her I didn't know if I could meet her every week. I said 'I want you to get another teacher because you're making such wonderful progress—I don't want you to lose it.' But she's persistent. She said, 'I don't care how long you take, *only you* will be my teacher.'"

It isn't hard to guess what richness this exchange must have given to Mrs. Kittner's life. Is there any greater satisfaction in life than being really needed?

APPARENTLY, PEOPLE WHO do good things tend to be pretty quiet about it—at least that's what I've found. But when I started looking for examples, suddenly, such people seemed to be all over the place.

One organization that is fairly well known, and that I have men-

Doing Good

tioned briefly before, is the Executive Job Corps, also known in some parts of the country as the Service Corps of Retired Executives (SCORE). They are retired men and women who volunteer their management expertise and experience to help younger people trying to start a business or, often, those who find themselves in serious difficulty, perhaps even facing the loss of their business and their means of making a living.

One such man had started a catering business, done very well with it, and then began rapid expansion with the aim of becoming a young millionaire. From the start, he had worked with the help of a member of SCORE, Bernard Splaver, a retired caterer who had a very successful catering-business career behind him. After retirement Mr. Splaver had joined the faculty of the Culinary Institute of America and, later, became its dean. Now, at seventy-seven, he works full-time for SCORE. The warning lights first went on for Splaver when he saw his would-be millionaire grab the lease on a newly vacated First National Store and plan to turn it into a restaurant to accompany the catering operation.

"I sat down with him," Splaver said, "and tried to make clear all the risks, and particularly, I warned him about the lease, a dangerously high thirty-five hundred dollars a month." But the young man ignored the advice, opened the restaurant, and tried to juggle the two businesses. As Splaver pointed out, these are businesses that each, by itself, calls for near-twenty-four-hours-a-day attention. And so it wasn't long at all before our young restaurateur-cum-caterer came back to Splaver with a long face. In a few words, he found himself up the well-known creek without the well-known paddle—in debt to the tune of $250,000, going further in every day—and impossible to live with at home. His family life was in serious jeopardy. His wife said he paced the floor all night, snapped at the children without cause, and appeared to have aged twenty years in a matter of months.

This was definitely a job for "Super-score," and Splaver jumped right in with both feet, determined to save his protégé if it was possible.

As Splaver told me this story, I could hear him actually reliving the battle in his tone of voice. It had been a challenge worthy of his skills and experience, and clearly, this seventy-seven-year-old young man's blood ran faster and life took on an intense meaning for him. Splaver spent days with the young caterer, trying to stave off creditors, get rid of the thirty-five-hundred-dollars-a-month drain, close the restaurant, and relocate the commissary in a low-rent situation. Also he told me, there was an important attitude change necessary. His protégé had leased a Mark III Lincoln Continental because he felt it was a good policy to serenade potential clients with the sweet smell of success. He would sweep up to their homes in his Continental, close the car door with that $20,000 "chunk" and walk in to discuss expenses of the wedding reception with the father of the bride, who, on seeing the car, probably thought, "So I'm going to have to help pay for that as well as everything else" and went back to the "yellow pages" for a caterer with a smaller ad.

As Splaver made this point, he said he told his young friend that he too had owned a Lincoln Continental—and an older Chevrolet. "When making a sales call," he said, "I always drove the Chevy." As so many Congressmen know, it's fine to have a Cadillac in Washington, but it's not a bad idea to tour the constituency at home in a Ford.

They got rid of the restaurant lease as soon as possible, found quarters for the commissary at $500 a month, and then ran a forecast on profitability under the new conditions. It looked good. But there remained a little problem of a quarter of a million dollars of debt and hungry, even angry, wholesale suppliers. It was here, perhaps, that Splaver made his greatest contribution. With his many years of experience, he was able to take the balance sheet and forecasts and tell a convincing story to the wholesalers, who were close to forcing the shaky catering business into bankruptcy. In addition, he suggested ways of amortizing the debts and worked closely with his protégé for more than a year. He also got right into the new kitchen and suggested how to redesign the space to make fewer steps for the employees, more efficient use of the area, and thus, one less employee. Today, only two years later, the debt has been reduced to $50,000! Also reduced is the caterer's blood pressure.

Doing Good

It struck me as quite a coincidence that at the time Splaver started work on reducing the quarter million of debt, he also discovered that he suffered from lymphoma, a serious form of cancer. But he's a busy man. As he put it, "Well, it has curtailed my activity a little bit. That is, after the chemotherapy treatments, I can't do too much for four or five days."

I asked Splaver why he ever got mixed up with the SCORE organization. "Well," he said, "I've always liked doing things for other people—my wife and I do a great deal of volunteer work, always have. I particularly like SCORE because it draws on my life's experience and, especially, because it lets me use those areas in which I'm strong. And I get a real kick out of it when somebody tells me I've helped them.

"Why, a young man came to me once and told me he wasn't making any money—just like that. He said his accountant had told him so. That's why he came to SCORE. So I told him to bring in his books, which he did, and we went over them with a fine-tooth comb. Almost right away I found $5,000 in inventory the accountant had missed completely. The man had tears in his eyes. In fact he was so grateful, he caught me by surprise—he bent right down and kissed me on the cheek! But it sure makes you feel good to know you've helped somebody along the way. And I'll tell you another reason why I like volunteer work—I never have to worry today about what I'm going to do tomorrow."

Bernard Splaver has given five years to SCORE so far, and it has not enriched him by five cents. But after hearing his story, is there any need to count the ways in which this man's life has been enlarged, the dimensions that have been added to it, the satisfactions that have been added to what might have been just one empty day after another? And I'm especially happy to be able to relate that Bernard Splaver's cancer, as of this writing, has been supressed.

The vast majority in medicine today are of the opinion that the mind and spirit exert untold influence over the condition of the body. For the past two years Myrtle Way, ninety-eight years old, has been teaching English to a seventy-year-old Russian immigrant. When the opportunity arose to take on her first student, Mrs. Way was thrilled. "I thought it was a worthwhile project," she said. Now Mrs. Way has recruited a new student, a Chinese woman who works in the dining room of the apartment complex where Way lives.

What would medicine have to say about the effect of Mrs. Way's good activities on her ninety-eight years? I'll leave you to draw your own conclusions.

OF COURSE, IT'S not necessary to belong to an organization to do good things for others. Irving Cohn is an eighty-six-year-old jeweler from Chicago, who works six days a week and is never happier than when selling diamond engagement rings to young couples. He's long past needing or wanting any more money, but he is quite convinced that his rings are lucky and that his couples will be, too. He whips a Polaroid camera out from under the counter and catches each couple right in the act of selecting their engagement ring. And it's incredible how pleased they seem to be when he presents them with the photograph.

Until a few years ago Cohn lived in the suburbs, on a dead-end street with a median divider running down the middle. He's the kind of man who spent a little time each week ensuring that the divider was bright with flowers during the summer months. But maybe the activity that characterizes him best is his membership in MOPH. I said he didn't belong to any organization, but MOPH is an exception. MOPH is an organization of one, namely Cohn, and its title stands for *Make Other People Happy*. As I said, this eighty-six-year-old works six days a week, but that still leaves him Sunday. And on Sundays, armed with his trusty Polaroid, Cohn sets out for a Chicago hospital.

What he does began with a visit to a sick friend, but now on Sundays, he roams the corridors looking for patients who appear lonely, sad, or just unloved. When he finds a likely target, he approaches and tries to engage the person in small talk. If they don't respond, he gives them a big smile and moves on. But the man is really a walking vaudeville act, and when he finds a patient who responds, who seems hungry for a little company, he goes to work.

Doing Good

He loves to tell outlandish, ridiculous stories, usually on himself. He's the first to admit that he's a clumsy man, always bumping into people and things. And one of his favorite stories is about the day his wife heard a deep thump downstairs and rushed into the recreation room in their home to find an astonished Cohn, sitting there—in his car! Entering the garage, he had missed the brake pedal and stepped on the accelerator.

Just when he is successful in bringing a little brightness or a smile into a patient's face, out comes the ever-present Polaroid, the smile is captured, and he delivers the evidence of the happy moment to the patient. "Leave 'em laughing" is the phrase in the theater. Leave 'em feeling good is what Cohn strives for. And that's what makes patients get well sooner; and that's what makes Irving Cohn's life rich and happy.

SOMETIMES WATCHING THE television news and reading the daily papers is a pretty depressing experience. Remember the picture of Justice, blindfolded and holding scales? If one of the weighing pans were marked "happiness" and the other, "misery," I'm sorely afraid misery would be on the lower side. But if enough of us were to toss something of ourselves onto the happiness side, it might redress the balance and, at the same time, give ourselves a better world to live in.

In speaking of his religion, Benjamin Franklin once described how he felt God should be served. "The most acceptable service we can render Him is to do good to His other children." One might well say of Arline Thomas, seventy-five, of Queens, New York that "her eye is on the sparrow" because Mrs. Thomas is a firm believer in Franklin's words on service to God, and she firmly includes her birds among "His other children."

Small and bright-eyed, Arline Thomas speaks rapidly and with such variety of tones and rhythms in her speech that I think she could have made quite a career on the stage. Injured birds have been her abiding interest for more than thirty years. Now a widow at seventy-five, Mrs. Thomas has an aviary attached to the outside of her house, where, at the moment, there are some fifteen birds at various stages of recovery. For more seriously damaged birds she has turned a part of her kitchen into what she calls the infirmary.

"Why the kitchen?" I asked her. And I got the feeling that she thought I might be somewhat retarded.

"For the refrigerator, of course," she replied. "When they first come in some of them have to be fed every few minutes." I told her about a mourning dove that had become entangled in a badminton net on my own back lawn and damaged its wings. Leaving it wrapped in a towel, I had run to call the local Audubon Society, but on my return, found its eyes glazed over in death.

"Shock," she said immediately. "With shock you must put the bird in a dark box, in a quiet place, and just leave it for two hours."

As we talked about the various aspects of running a bird hospital, I realized that these activities filled almost all of Mrs. Thomas's day. I wondered how it had all started. After all, no woman starts out at the age of forty to care for birds so that she'll be busy and feel useful when she's a widow thirty-five years later. "How did it begin?" I asked.

"With a one-eyed nuthatch," she replied.

She told me how she and her husband had set up a bird feeder simply for the pleasure of seeing the different varieties. "Then," she said, "a little nuthatch came, and we got to know him because he had only one eye. He'd come to the window and he'd yell, 'Ank, ank!' I found that he loved peanuts. We fed him all winter and then, in March, he disappeared.

"One day, I was working in the garden when I noticed this gray thing crawling along—I thought it was a mouse. Then I saw it was our little nuthatch, with the one eye, and it seemed to recognize me and came crawling to me. So I took him into the kitchen because I knew what to feed him, his favorite peanuts. I fixed up a box, with a garden sieve over the top and a stick to perch on. He had somehow sprained one wing and simply couldn't fly. But after three weeks of nothing more than gentle care, he was flying around the kitchen, and I was able to let him go. He just flew up into one of the big oak trees and that was it."

"Do you ever keep any birds?" I asked.

Doing Good

"Nope," was the decisive reply. "And I've never named a bird because I don't want to get emotionally attached. As I see it the birds come here (or are brought here now in many cases) to get their health back. It's my job to enable them to return to the wild—not to make pets out of them."

So here is Mrs. Thomas, a widow, seventy-five years old, living alone and yet living a far richer life than that of many others who seem superficially better situated. "It's very fulfilling," she says. "And it certainly does keep you busy. I get an injured seagull, and the first thing I have to do is run out and buy fish."

I want to give the last words in this chapter to Mrs. Thomas—"You get what you give in this life."

7

Winds of Change

We must cut our coat according to our cloth.
—Lylly

We've done some speculating about when life begins, in this book, from various points of view. About when LIFE, in capitals, actually began, we know precious little. Maybe a stray cosmic ray struck something down in the primeval ooze that was just itching to get started. An ooze-age chemical reaction took place. Millions of years later, something wiggled. A few million more years later, something swam. A few million years after that the swimming thing flopped out of the water, probably in a tidal pool, and moved a little on the land. With no scientific basis, I feel that these wiggling, swimming, flopping, and finally walking things did so because they wanted to! I can safely say this because I will make no attempt to prove it. And I have to say it for myself because I can find no other way to explain the miraculous acts of adaptation that have been accomplished by living creatures down through the millions of years of evolution. In fact, this ability to adapt appears to have been the key to survival for the myriads of forms of life on earth. We all know how the lamented dinosaur failed the test of adaptability to some great climactic or other change a few million years ago and, equally, how man has nimbly adapted to the challenges he faced. Once he really began to use his brain, he was freed from the evolutionary process and

LIFE BEGINS AT SIXTY

began to use such tools as fire, artificial shelter, clothing, central heating, rockets, and artificial atmospheres. Now he can exist anywhere on earth and even on the moon, if he wants to.

So also as individuals we've had plenty of experience adapting as we matured. With trepidation we first left home and walked or were bussed to school. We went with fear and trembling to our first big dance, and from high school or college out to the work scene. Later, we adapted to little people screaming all night and spilling food on our clothes. Some years later, we left the work scene. Now, in our mature years, every bit of our skill at adapting is going to be called for. The changes we will face are greater than any that have gone before and often irreversible. We may find ourselves forced to live on without a beloved spouse. We'll likely have to adapt to making do with less money. We may hear or see less acutely. If we hit a lottery, we may have to adapt to living with astronomically unfamiliar amounts of money. Don't laugh; many have failed that challenge ignominiously.

So the necessity of adapting to some pretty important changes is usually the biggest thing facing us as we move into the third period, sixty to ninety-plus years. Fortunately the people of our generation, those of us whose lives span the twentieth century, are peculiarly suited to handling the challenge. Never in the entire history of mankind has any group of people seen such radical change in their lifetime as we have.

A life that was based on agriculture and that had lasted ten thousand years or more, came to an end during the last century. All of us born between 1890 and 1920 have lived with the most rapid change and stress humankind has ever seen. In the material world, almost all the gadgets that seem to fill our lives today came into use after we were born. Automobiles, telephones, airplanes, dishwashers, television, personal computers simply didn't exist around the time of our birth. Even the radio of my childhood was a crystal set I had sent away for. We scratched that little needle around on the surface of the crystal until suddenly, in the earphones, the faint voice of KDKA in Pittsburgh came through to upstate New York.

"Adapt or die," that's the challenge. But let's not get melodramatic about it. Maybe "Adapt or be miserable" is more like it. I recently

Winds of Change

talked about the subject of adapting with an 80-year-old who has spent most of his life studying human behavior, Dr. B. F. Skinner of Harvard. He told me of a number of changes he has made with advancing years simply because, as he put it, "The old way of doing things didn't pay off anymore." Something as simple as going out to dinner at a restaurant with friends had changed. Usually, the more chic the restaurant, the darker, and Skinner has glaucoma and doesn't see as well as formerly. "So when I get there," he said, "I can't read the menu. I can hardly see or understand the person across the table. When they take my plate away, I find I've pushed the food off the plate and there it lies on the table." His conclusion: "I shouldn't go to dark restaurants anymore."

Many of the changes that call for adapting are equally simple. Strangely, many of us have more trouble with the little things than the large. Unlike our friend, Reynolds Wait, who regularly tore up the road between Skaneatles, New York, and his furniture stores until the age of ninety, Dr. Skinner has given up driving because of his poor eyesight.

The problem, as he describes it, is not moving out of the driver's seat but moving out of the driver's mentality—of restraining himself from being "co-pilot." "So," Skinner said, "my wife usually drives me. For fifty-odd years, I've watched the road ahead, watched traffic lights (Are they going to turn before we get there? Are cars coming out from side streets?), and so on. None of that is useful anymore," Skinner stated with more cool detachment than I could have mustered. "But it's hard to stop it. I've slowly learned to look out of the window and look at other things. If I can't do that, I just look down. I do not look ahead anymore. *You just have to learn,*" he said very firmly. "You practice it. I found it difficult. It took me some time."

There, I think, Skinner has given us the recipe for change. And although these examples have to do with simple, less than earthshaking changes, I believe they will apply equally to the great changes and the major adaptations we may be called upon to make.

SALLY MCINTOSH, NOW eighty-one, has had a lot of adapting to do in recent years. "Keep busy" has been her motto all her life. And she has certainly done so since, in Detroit in 1932, she started the first radio program devoted to what women do outside of the home. "As I was first planning the content of the program, I spent some time listening to other women's programs, which dealt with decorating, cooking, sewing, and all that. I still remember my mother's look of shocked astonishment when I said, 'You know that's all a lot of crap.' And I did a show that dealt with what women did in a man's world."

From a five-days-a-week radio program, McIntosh moved on to reporting on consumer affairs, then to the Consumer Affairs Department for General Mills. At that job she met Mabel Flanley, who did the same for the Borden Company. They got together and started Flanley and Woodward, Public Relations. Sally Woodward had been McIntosh's "stage name" for the radio program. Flanley and Woodward prospered for years until Flanley decided to retire, and they sold the company.

Now, change struck in the form of idle time. Sally McIntosh had always been a busy person. Then one day, she looked at her calendar and there was nothing on it. "It was an unexpected shock," she said, "but thankfully, it shocked me into doing something. I made up my mind then that I wouldn't go to bed at night unless I had a project for the next day. It might be something as mundane as dreaded mending or some writing or even cleaning a closet—but it was there for me to start in on as soon as I finished my tea in the morning."

Another change to which Sally McIntosh has had to adapt is the onset of arthritis. "My arthritis has thrown my hip out and stooped my shoulders badly. Every time I look in the mirror, that's a change I can't get used to. I don't like what I see. I remember when the boys turned around and looked." She laughed. "Well, now, they probably don't look much better than I do." Throughout the interview Sally's sense of humor came into play. "I used to do a great deal of traveling. Now, it's five years since the arthritis made me stop. But what I do about that is I travel vicariously. I have two large atlases and everything that happens—I have to look it up and visualize just where it's all going on. I drive the AAA crazy because I buy so many maps.

Sally also has friends all over the world, and she keeps in touch. "I

Winds of Change

want to be interested in them rather than them calling up and saying, 'Well, Sally, how are you getting along?' I'll call people at the drop of a hat. It costs a lot less than traveling. I try to think of it that way." Even so Sally was surprised at how many people she is actually in regular touch with. She'll be moving into a new apartment soon. "Now that I'm moving, I wrote a round-robin letter and I had ninety-eight people to send it to."

Later, Sally used an expression I'd never heard before when she said, "I'm not first to anybody." It sounds a little sad, doesn't it? Most of us, including Sally, go through life being "first to somebody"—parent, husband, wife—and yet the time comes, if we live long enough, when we find we are not first to anybody. If we can find it in our capacity to accept that fact as another aspect of life, then, we will also be able to gain great satisfaction and happiness from being "second to many."

A few years ago, Sally got involved with Literacy Volunteers of America. She helps people for whom English is a second language to improve their skills in order to get along better in day-to-day living. For the past year Sally has been working with a young woman from India, who is married to a man employed as an engineer for a well-known American firm. Since "Literacy Volunteers" are usually senior citizens, the student goes to the home of the volunteer teacher twice a week. When she first started, Sally's student couldn't handle a checkbook and could barely shop for her family. Now, one year later, the young Indian woman shops with ease, handles the family's accounts, and even holds down a six-to-ten job as cashier in a pharmacy. She and Sally McIntosh may not be first to each other but they are surely close seconds.

AT THIS POINT, I'd like to bring up another change that overtakes most of us sooner or later. To do so, come back with me to England in the winter of 1945, toward the end of World War II. I was a pilot then, flying for the U.S. Army Air Corps. One cold night in February, with no flight scheduled for the next day, I spent the evening with an English girl with whom I was very much in love. It was late, her parents were upstairs in bed, and we were sitting in front of a warm fire in the living room. It was a quiet time. She was curled up in my lap and we were staring into the fire. I finally said what I had come there to say that night. "How would you like to spend the rest of your life with me?" That was forty years ago. We were married the following June and lived happily ever after.

But, and this is a big "but," there is a good chance that one of us will have to live the last years of life alone. How can one adapt to that kind of change? The truth is that some cannot. The broken heart is not only a poetic fancy, it is a medical reality.

One medical authority told me that "there's a lot of evidence that the number of people who die within one year of their spouse's death is outrageously high—it's something like two to three times as much as one would expect from statistics. We don't know exactly the reasons: whether people just give up the will to live, whether there are certain—you know some people just go out and become alcoholic, something like that. Or sometimes it's like two people helping each other physically to maintain their medication—one is physically helping the other in a way that when one is lost, a certain support system is lost. But I think that's quite separate from a loss of the will to live."

Mary LeCain of Melbourne, Florida, now seventy-six, lost her husband two years ago. As she said, "He was sitting there in a chair with a group of us talking, and then, suddenly, he was gone." Now she's alone a great deal of the time, and her loneliness is typified by incidents like the following. "I may be sitting there watching television and see something especially interesting. I'll turn to say something to my husband—and he's not there. It just hits you like that." Yet Mrs. LeCain has overcome the problem of loneliness, and she's done it by a conscious effort of will. "I've seen friends," she said, "who feel sorry for themselves and make themselves miserable. I just made up my mind not to be like those others."

Mrs. LeCain first developed an affection for her husband when they were both in the sixth grade. It lasted sixty-two years, until his death; so she can barely remember a time when they were not together. But having "made up my mind" as she put it, she took a number of distinct actions to meet loneliness head on. She lives in Florida during the winter months, in a comfortable trailer she and her husband bought some years ago. It's permanently stationed in a well-run trailer park, and although she is alone, she is near a great many friends she and her husband knew together. The residents built a recreation hall, formed an organized group, and so all sorts of activities are available. Mrs. LeCain makes a point of taking classes there and also at a local senior center where she lives in the North during the summer. Continuing education is an important part of her life.

THERE IS AN active senior citizens center in the town where I live. As a result of shrinking school enrollment, typical of the Northeast today, a full wing of an unused school is now set aside by the town for the center. I drop in now and then to meet people and attend some functions. Last week, the director of the center asked me if I would like to go into New York with a group of recent high school graduates for a tour of *The New York Times* and the United Nations. Puzzled, I asked her, "Why do I want to go to New York with a bunch of high school kids?"

"Well, most of them are in their seventies," she replied. I was amazed. Some twenty or thirty men and women had attended classes given at the center and completed their education, receiving high school diplomas. Now they were going on "their class trip" just as I remember my children doing. Of course, I went with them.

Now, two days later, my back has yet to recover from the bone-crushing, three-hour ride in the school bus. It made me wonder if we're not damaging our children's kidneys with such primitive transportation. But the trip was great. The noise level, chatter, and laughter in that bus would be hard to distinguish from when it is carrying the kids. The "students" were a perfect example of what happens to people who set out to satisfy their curiosity and take part in interesting activities.

We all piled out at the Forty-Second Street entrance to the Times Building and were taken by a competent guide through the editorial floors: sports, business, politics, foreign affairs, restaurant and drama critics—could I have missed literary critics?—and other special sections. We went to the basement to see the mammoth presses that are set into the bedrock under New York because their vibration when running would otherwise actually damage nearby buildings. Each one of these three-million-dollar machines turns out, in one hour, fifty-five thousand finished, four-section, completely collated papers just like the one that lands on my front porch! We marveled at the "laser room," with danger signs everywhere saying "dangerous visible and invisible laser beams." From here, I was astounded to learn, the computer typesetting tapes containing the entire day's national edition are beamed up to a satellite twenty-four thousand miles above the earth and thence down to Dallas, California, and Chicago, where they accomplish the typesetting of the next day's edition.

Next we entered the editorial conference room, where weighty decisions on the *Times*'s editorial stance are taken, and enjoyed a forty-five-minute meeting with the columnist Russell Baker. His book *Growing Up* had been a graduation gift to each student.

Of course, each wanted Baker's book autographed, and as I watched them take their copies in turn, saying a few words and looking at him in admiration, it struck me that they were, in effect, so much like teenage high school students that virtually the only difference was in appearance. They talked like students, their expressions looked like students—well, I suddenly realized, they *were* students. One little lady, a platinum blond with marcelled hair and all of four feet ten inches, looked up in awe at Russell Baker's six feet-plus while he signed her book. The experience she was going through, what she felt at that moment, had to be no different from that of a young high school girl.

CURIOSITY SEEMS TO have been the motive for the members of this lively group to return to their education and earn their high school diplomas in their seventies. As a motive, curiosity has been among mankind's most rewarding drives. It has been said that necessity was the mother of invention. If so, curiosity was almost certainly the father.

Curiosity about where he came from led Alex Haley to years of research about his ancestors until he finally found his "roots" in Africa, wrote a best-selling book and television miniseries, and suddenly found himself a very wealthy man.

You may think I'm taking a very roundabout approach to my next subject, but there are some who would dismiss it by saying "Don't ever look back, something may be gaining on you." I say, nonsense. Looking back can be very pleasurable when taken in moderation. We often hear, "She lives in the past," said in a pejorative manner. But it can be very pleasurable to relive former victories and remember the sunny days of our youth. Perhaps, we should take the Roman god Janus as our model. You remember he is depicted as having two bearded faces, one looking ahead and the other looking backward. Janus, god of doorways and gates, would tell us that there is no harm in looking back as long as we also live in the present and look with a lively interest to the future.

So now I've finally come to my subject, and it is *looking back*. As Sally McIntosh one day looked at her calendar and found nothing on it, so all of us have periods when there is nothing on the calendar. I am recommending an occupation that can be fascinating for you and, perhaps, even more fascinating for your children and grandchildren. It has the potential for filling days and months of your time with surprises, colorful facts about your past, characters who played their own roles in shaping some part of our history, and a great part of your own history. You know, of course, that I'm talking about genealogy, the story of your descent from ancestors both recent and ancient. I've always believed that a sense of identity is basic to living our lives with purpose and satisfaction. I'm not talking about trying to prove we are related to the queen of England or descended from ancient Italian nobility. I'm talking about finding out who of our forebears first came to this continent, and, perhaps, how they came and why. Where did they come from in Germany, Scotland, England, or Africa? What knowledge and skills did they bring with them? What tragedies, noble moments, or victories were the high points of their lives? This is knowledge that can amuse, please, or even sadden you. In a very real sense it is a part of your past—a part of what shaped you. And remember, it is all those things and perhaps even more to your children and grandchildren.

Most important of all, this is an area where you are indispensable. No matter how close you may be with your children, there is a massive amount of knowledge in your head that they simply know nothing about. I've mentioned my grandmother before, the one who was born in 1857 and lived to 1952. Since I was lucky enough to know her for thirty-two years, we had many conversations. And since I was always curious. I managed to prise many stories from her. There was the exciting tale of her honeymoon when, in 1878, she and my grandfather went to California in a stagecoach—it was a risky business in those days. Only two years before, General Custer had died at Little Big Horn. Even more interesting to me, she remembered snatches from before and during the Civil War; the hunger, the shortages, and soldiers' stories. And in her childhood there were still people alive who had seen George Washington.

I mentioned all the things in your memory that your children don't know exist. There's probably a lot there that you don't know about either. And beyond what you know yourself, there are clues and leads to more and more information—stories that would enrich the lives of your descendants. It's unfortunate that keeping family history alive often is of little interest to children and young adults. I've noticed this with my own children. It wasn't until they got into their middle or late thirties that they began to ask questions about family and the past.

So I'm suggesting that one of those days when you find your "calendar" with nothing on it, you start on a little detective project. It can keep you just as busy as you want. The search will call for initiating some or a lot of correspondence. It will take as many telephone calls or visits as you care to make. In some cases, if you are well-fixed financially and want to spend the time, it can call for moderate or extensive travel. But to start, all you need is paper and a

Winds of Change

ball point pen. Starting with your parents and grandparents, go back as far as you can, writing the names in a "V" with your name at the bottom. Without complicating things unduly, you can fill out a small card for each person, listing dates, where born, and any other information you may think interesting. The questions will begin to pile up rapidly; some you'll want to find the answers to very much—others you'll forget. For example, one of my grandmothers came from Ireland in the 1880s to work as a kitchen maid in my great grandfather's house. Before that, her origin is a complete mystery. I would love to know something about it. In a way her story is typically American. Beginning in the kitchen she had become, by the time of my last clear memory of her, the "grande dame" with pink cheeks, blue eyes, and a cloud of white hair—presiding over my sister's "coming out" party at the St. Regis Roof in New York just before World War II. Where did she come from before boarding that ship in Queenstown on Ireland's south coast? I'll probably never know. Yet if I had asked the questions, or if she had thought to write a few facts down... well, the chance has passed forever.

Another mystery in my family concerns my great Uncle Howard who died in Lancaster, England, in 1898, at the age of thirty-seven. Uncle Howard was a bon vivant on two continents, as they used to say. I once found a clipping from a Paris newspaper in the 1890s reporting that Howard Case and a friend hosted a grande fete for two thousand guests in the Bois de Boulogne. It described the lights in the trees, the names of well-known guests, the music, and so on. The fact that he "lived it up" was well known in the family; and also known was the fact that he died in Lancaster while on a coaching trip. But there were many rumors. I heard that he'd been murdered by his valet or had a sudden heart attack or that he succumbed to an overdose of cocaine. In those days cocaine was thought to be harmless.

Once, an old and good friend of the family said to me about Howard; "Oh, that's a really terrible story, Billy. Maybe some day, I'll tell you about it." Unfortunately, I didn't insist, and now, he's been dead for years. A newspaper clipping that I have states that it was a heart attack. But another from an English paper says that the inquest was hurried and that many members of the coroner's jury thought that a fuller investigation should have taken place. Shades of English detective novels.

A couple of years ago my wife and I visited her relatives in Lancashire, where she was born. On the way to Scotland to visit other relatives, we passed through Lancaster with its great twelfth-century Norman castle brooding on a hill. Unfortunately, the "Old Country Hotel" where Uncle Howard died, almost ninety years ago, is no longer there—so another mystery will never be solved. If I or anyone in the family had done what I recommend you do, the story would be complete and would become one of the old family tales to be passed along by my children.

Have I piqued your curiosity at all about your own forebears? I surely hope so. And I hope you spend many fulfilling and interesting hours "detecting" among letters, newspaper clippings, old wills, and other documents and, especially, communicating with other members of the family, near and far, in the quest for knowledge of, and interesting stories about, your roots. And for the sake of your descendants, don't forget to write it down.

"CONTINUING EDUCATION"—on the face of it that's a pretty boring phrase. How about "further exploration" into all the magical things that are going on all around us—and have been going on for centuries? A short while back, we saw a group of seventy-year-olds earning their high school diplomas. Now, I want to tell you about a retired professional man who is taking advantage of an organization set up specifically for people of somewhat advanced education and accomplishments. His name is David Burke, and he is retired and sixty-seven years old—a youngster for this book, but he is qualified. Shortly, he will be starting his third year studying at an unusual organization, the Institute for Retired Professionals (IRP).

The IRP was set up as a cooperative venture between the Department of Aging of the town of Fairfield, Connecticut, and Fairfield University. In the words of David Burke: "It is for people who have broad interests and a desire for continuing education. One of the clues is that a person who reads a lot will like this program or the symposia as they are called. The subjects of these seminars are varied, very eclectic, and appeal to a great breadth in interests and talents.

"At eighty dollars per semester I think the institute's programs are the greatest education buy of the century," Burke said. "You'll go from subjects like the history of the English novel to the historical intrusions of the Soviet Union into the Middle East to the development and manufacture of the Hubble telescope." (The latter will be part of the payload on a shuttle mission scheduled for early 1986.)

"How often are these symposia held?" I asked.

"Once a month," Burke replied, "but membership in the Institute for Retired Professionals goes far beyond that. For example, they have special interest groups. I took the one held last year on 'Religion in America,' four sessions, and these come under the same eighty dollars. There were about twenty of us in that course."

Burke's enthusiasm was clear in his voice. His own background is at the executive level in the General Electric Company. Among other responsibilities, he was producer on the company side of the "General Electric Theater," famous television series back in the "Golden Years" of TV. Obviously, the change that retirement meant to his responsibilities and intellectual life was massive. But he has chosen to adapt in varied ways. He is also an accomplished artist, but the IRP arouses the most enthusiasm in him.

"Another great thing," he said, "is that you have the opportunity to participate in the university's continuing education program. Here are courses, leading to degrees, attended by people in their thirties, forties, fifties, and even sixties. And we who are enrolled in the Institute for Retired Professionals can take any of the courses on an audit basis."

Burke described a field trip symposium that Martha Plotkin, director of the Fairfield Department on Aging, has organized for the coming year. Physicians of the cardiac unit of nearby Bridgeport Hospital will be hosts at a luncheon for the students, followed by a tour of the unit, conducted by the physician in charge.

"What's really appealing about this program," Burke said, "Is the great breadth of the courses. And when you take a class as an auditor you can participate just as far as you want—even up to taking the exams. I find I can't participate in a class without going through the whole drill. When I asked the professor if I could take the examination, he was a little surprised. But I took it. Frankly, I was a little curious if my brain was up to it." He paused a moment thoughtfully. "I have to tell you I was a little discouraged by the results. I didn't come up to the mark as well as I might have."

Then Burke told me how he had told his wife about the exam results: "'Well, what can you expect,' I said, 'I'm getting older.' But she didn't let me get away with that for a minute." She had said that, according to what is known today, the brain and our intelligence continue to grow right into the eighties and nineties. And the lady is absolutely right. Current research reveals continued growth in the capacity of our brains, illness aside of course, virtually as long as we live.

There is great variety in the makeup of the Institute for Retired Professionals, Burke told me. "We have doctors, dentists, business people—about as many women as men—yes, a great variety of professions, occupations, and interests." I can hardly think of a better way to keep the mind supple than becoming active in a group like that.

The ability to adapt—one of mankind's greatest strengths for survival—is one you have to be aware of, and make use of, during the "living" years. A sneaky thing about it is that changes calling for adaptation on your part often take place so slowly and subtly that you may be unaware of them. Take impaired hearing as an example. The loss of sharp hearing can take place so slowly over a period of years that one simply doesn't notice it. And the reaction will often be, "People just don't speak clearly anymore, do they?" Then the person with fading hearing will find they like (or need) the television turned up a little bit louder than anyone else. A clue might be having neighbors complain about the volume of the radio or the TV. In any case one solution is simple. Buy a pair of glasses with the hearing device built right into the frames. Remember the visit to *The New York Times* with those septuagenarian high school students? When

Winds of Change

Russell Baker, the columnist, spoke to us in the conference room, he said that he first had to put on his glasses—not to see us with, but to hear us with. After he had them in place no one would have imagined that he didn't hear as well as the rest of us.

Somebody once said (I can't remember them all) that the "solution of a problem is always inherent in a clear statement of it." If there is a problem in your life that calls for adapting on your part, articulate it as clearly as you can. Discuss it with a friend or mentor at length. Talk all around it. Identify the change in your environment that is making you uncomfortable. Then, when what is bothering you is quite clear, devise whatever kind of adapting on your part is necessary to make you comfortable again. Use friends, your physician, or anyone else who might be able to help. But above all use the God-given ability of the human race to adapt.

8

Variety

The very spice of life that gives it all its flavor.
—William Cowper

Variety is the subject of Cowper's lines, and those who live without it live in a gray, unchanging world that is the antithesis of life. *Variety* is the name of the bible of the world of show business, and variety, itself, is still an absolute must in the worlds of the theater, movies, and television. The other day, I went along with a troupe of variety artists to enjoy their performance for a group of old and infirm people in a nursing home. Making up the troupe were a pianist, a violinist, a girl singer, a couple of comedians, and various other performers. As I joined the group and we arrived at the home, I was reminded of the special atmosphere that exists among entertainers. It's a mixture of camaraderie, nervous tension before "going on," and the humor everybody projects to relieve that tension. The noise level is pretty high, the jokes fly fast and furious, and there is that special ego-flattering feeling of being the center of attention. The fact is that whether you are playing an instrument, singing, or doing a comedy skit, you are placing yourself at the mercy of an audience. It's fun and scary at the same time.

When we arrived, some patients were awaiting us in the large, cleared dining room, and others were still being wheeled in. The first thing to do in any show is to get the attention of the audience and get them on your side. So the troupe started with a sing-along, taking requests from the audience and securing their participation right from the start. Then they began the show itself. Wearing straw boaters with bright ribbons, they paraded around the room, first humming and then bursting into the favorite "One of Those Shows." Then came the solos: a blue-eyed beauty belted out "Ma, He's Makin' Eyes at Me" to applause and smiles; a black-haired soprano crooned "You're Always on My Mind"; a tall, lanky baritone gave a full-throated rendition of "I Believe," made even more moving by his expressionless face; and then, in a break from singing, two men sat, holding newspapers, and exchanging some of the worst, tired jokes I've heard in years. They were so bad, they were hilarious; and the audience laughed both at and with the performers.

Then, in a change of pace, the troupe leader asked the audience for their ages. At first, they were slow to volunteer; then a husky female voice said, "I'm seventy-eight." "Just a child," said the leader. Another piped up with an "eighty-one." After each age was announced, there was applause. A white-haired lady with blue eyes and pink cheeks shouted, "Eighty-six." More applause. Then a slightly cracked man's voice called out, "Ninety-one," followed by the loudest applause of all; and I guess he was the winner.

Finally, after more sing-alongs, they announced the finale. The whole troupe joined hands for "Goodnight, Goodnight," swaying right and left and then easing into "Auld Lang Syne." The patients were mesmerized, eyes glued on the performers, usually concentrating on their favorite as most of us do—and those eyes became a little teary at the end. Once the show was over, the troupe stood around in knots, chatting with the nurses and the director of the home and drinking punch, which was provided for all. The patients, almost all in wheelchairs, kept their eyes on the performers as the first patient was wheeled slowly out.

Just then an anonymous voice started the words to "America the Beautiful." Some of the others hummed; more joined in. Another voice then slipped into "Amazing Grace," that gently moving spiritual, and again almost everyone's lips were moving. It appeared that

Variety

nobody wanted to leave. Then the baritone, with his full voice, started that almost majestic musical version of "Our Father." As he soared with "Who art in heaven," the troupe joined more vigorously. The volume built until I felt engulfed in waves of sound. "For thine is the kingdom..." The room vibrated with sound and we were all part of it; there was a oneness I cannot describe. And then it was over. Good-byes all around and the troupe prepared to leave.

Did I mention that the troupers' ages ran from sixty, the singer, to eighty-six, the soprano who sang "Ma, He's Makin' Eyes...?" The pianist was eighty-one; the violinist, seventy-six; an average age of probably around eighty. Good troupers all, they had given a couple of hours of escape to those patients—escape from unending pain, from living in the darkness of the totally blind, from a loneliness that numbs the mind, and for most of them, from living a passive life. After the entertainers left, the patients would talk for days about the little incidents that made up the performance. Yet it is difficult to say who, patients or performers, got the most out of it. Paraphrasing Portia in *The Merchant of Venice*, the show was twice blessed; it blessed those who gave, and it blessed those who received.

Later when I had the opportunity, I asked the members of the troupe what motivated them to give so much of their time to rehearsing and traveling around to put on shows like the one I had seen. "It makes a change," was one thing they all said. "It's one way of getting out of the house," one said, with a somewhat sardonic laugh. "I like going to the different places where we sing," said another. "It's a different experience every time." What they were all saying was that the shows brought variety into their lives.

TAKE AN INVENTORY of your own skills and talents. Do you sing, act, tell jokes well, play an instrument? Be honest with yourself, we're not looking for Eddy Duchins here or Laurence Oliviers or Buddy Hacketts—just talents that are a couple of levels above none. If the answer is "Yes," go join a group. Just try it once.

Oh, of course, you don't know of such a group. You've never heard of one where you live. Be advised there is one—almost certainly. Is there a senior citizens center or a convalescent home anywhere near you? Visit or telephone and ask; you will almost certainly get the names of those who do a little entertaining. If you don't want to telephone and volunteer yourself, just arrange casually to meet them at the senior center. I guarantee that once you have shown interest, you'll be asked to lend your talent.

Don't underestimate your power to entertain. If I learned anything from watching that troupe, it was the power of "live" entertainment. Those people weren't all that talented, and down the hall there were somewhat better singers and actors to be seen in the television room. Yet the TV room was empty. Why? Because those people were performing solely for those in that room. And because of that, some kind of two-way communication springs up between performers and viewers. And that communication is unique and beautiful in a way that television's one-way street never can be.

HERE'S ANOTHER DECEPTIVELY simple way of bringing a bit of variety into your routine. Do you have some place you walk to once a week or so?—the library? a grocery store? And have you found the shortest way of getting there and back? Do you use that route regularly? Next time change it. Start walking along different streets and turning where you've never turned before. Make the trip longer, unless you're carrying heavy packages. And if you go by car, make it longer anyway. Be on the lookout for new sights and new experiences, and let your curiosity run rampant. Ask yourself what kind of people live in the dwellings you pass. Look for clues in the gardens, in the condition of the buildings. Are there children outside? Pets? What vehicles are visible, and what do they suggest about the owners? Like a good detective, keep your eyes peeled for anything that could have meaning. And when you get home, test your memory by trying to list everything you saw. Talk about it and tell whomever you live with what you saw and what you deduced.

I'm trying to make you into a first-class gossip. After all, there's little that's more entertaining than flavorful gossip, and no harm done without intent, which you surely won't have. If you live alone,

Variety

try writing down notes on all the new things you saw. Use them to jog your memory for talking to a friend at a later time.

Let's not let variety run rampant throughout your entire life, however. Some routine, like always keeping kitchen implements in the same place, is a way of making life more simple. After all, if you had to invent anew how to tie the knots in your shoelaces every day, it would take a long time to get dressed.

Let's say you have a routine of doing your food shopping for the week Tuesday morning around half past ten. The market is nearly empty at that time, and you can get the job done twice as quickly as it would take on a Saturday; that's a good routine to keep. But let's say you watch the six o'clock news on the same television station every day. Break your routine tomorrow and pick a different time and station. Sample the different ones for a few days and make yourself a critic. Note what segments of the different programs are better than others: sports, weather, local news, national and international news. After a week or so, you'll be ready to do your review. But a review is no good if nobody reads it. So you must write it, and you must send it where it will do the most good—to the station you are critiquing.

When I was around ten years old, my parents sent me away to a boarding school; a change in my young life that I certainly did not welcome. While it was not a harsh school in the Dickensian sense, it might be considered a little tough today. Religion was part of the schedule, of course; and the choice of the hymn always sung on the first night back at school still puzzles me. It contained the line; "The night is dark and we are far from home." Tears were not far from most young eyes.

But what I want to talk about is food. It was excellent, as I remember. The only thing wrong with it was that it was boring. Apparently, the dietician had planned twenty-one meals once and then departed. Every meal given at a particular time of day on a particular day of the week was the same throughout the year. For me that was some fifty-four years ago, and I still remember some of the menus. Friday night was always codfish balls (the school was in Massachusetts), and Saturday noon was baked beans on toast. Maybe they figured it was best to give us beans on a day when we wouldn't be sitting cooped up in classrooms. Anyway the point is that it was pretty dull to know exactly what you were going to have for dinner a week from Wednesday and two weeks from Wednesday and . . . Yet I'm surprised to find that a lot of people just slip into that routine without thinking much about it. Have you?

Dr. Skinner says it is necessary to make deliberate changes. Here's one way to do that. Every newspaper, magazine, and Sunday supplement contains food recipes. Start cutting out ones that interest you and keep them in a little box or in a kitchen drawer. Then, before you go food shopping, run through them and take the one you fancy with you so you'll remember the ingredients. This isn't quite as stupid as it sounds because if you don't take it step by step, you'll never end up with variety in your menus. Obviously, these suggestions are not for the adventurous, gourmet cooks but, rather, for those who have inadvertently slipped into a rut gastronomically speaking. Incidentally, you'll be taking an important step toward good nutrition when you follow this advice. A broad variety of foods is the easiest way of making sure you get all the minerals and vitamins your body needs.

Another kind of beneficial variety was recommended by Benjamin Franklin. Dr. Franklin, who certainly ought to know, said something to the effect that travel may not make you live longer, but it makes life seem longer. And isn't it true that three weeks spent traveling in Europe feels like a much bigger piece of your life than three ordinary weeks at home? Travel can be one of the most pleasurable ways of bringing variety into your life. The effect is much the same whether you spend thousands on a fifteen-day cruise on the *Queen Elizabeth 2* in the Caribbean, or $399 for a week in Las Vegas "air fare included." The anticipation, new clothes (bought or made) different food, new faces, places that arouse your curiosity, and constant stimulation that makes you look ten years younger—not only do they tend to make you live longer, they make life more worth living.

You awaken one morning to find your great ship at anchor more than a mile outside the harbor of St. Thomas in the Virgin Islands. Peering out of the porthole you see the sparkling waves, brilliant

Variety

sunshine, and little bright flashes from the sun glinting off the cars at the distant harborside. Why so distant? You learn at breakfast. The size of your ship is so great that she cannot enter the harbor. You will be going ashore in launches that will spend the day ferrying passengers between the ship and St. Thomas.

Or you board your jet at La Guardia Airport, and fifteen minutes later, breakfast is being served as you climb smoothly toward the West, catching only a glimpse of the Hudson River and Pennsylvania sliding smoothly below. Two thirds of the country passes beneath you; the broad grasslands of the Midwest. With luck your pilot may show you the Grand Canyon and, then, the emptiness of vast deserts as you plane down to the Las Vegas airport and bus in and check into your hotel.

Or you wake from the three hour night that characterizes the 8:15 P.M. British Airways flight from New York to London. The captain announces that you are descending over Cornwall and Devonshire, and a moment later, he points out Windsor Castle as you swing northeast over the Thames and suddenly that one-time target of the Nazi bombers moves slowly underneath and you spot the Houses of Parliament and the Tower of London. A gentle bump on the runway at Heathrow and you are in the land of William the Conqueror, Anne Boleyn, and Princess Diana.

The problem with the foregoing is that such thoughts frighten a lot of people. You may not be one of them, but too many people feel immediately uneasy at the thought of leaving the safe, familiar nest and well-known routine that is home. It costs too much. I might get sick. What if I run out of money? I won't know anybody. And so on. Yet if you turn your back on the healthy variety that travel can bring to your life, you'll be missing one of the major pleasures that the freedom of age offers. People who are not tied down to regular jobs enjoy the opportunity of traveling when others can't.

VIOLA DOLZANI, SIXTY-SEVEN, has become a confirmed travel buff since she was widowed nine years ago, and she doesn't spend a fortune on her globe-trotting. So far, she has found two excellent sources of travel

LIFE BEGINS AT SIXTY

ideas at a reasonable cost: her local senior citizens center and travel agencies that advertise "specials" (some for seniors and others for groups of any age). Two of her recent trips were an agency-planned special to Las Vegas for six days and another senior citizen-planned bus trip to the World's Fair in Tennessee. The Las Vegas trip cost $399, including air fare, hotel, and some meals. The Tennessee trip cost $549, including motel and meals.

I asked Mrs. Dolzani how many trips she made this year. "Well, this year only one," she said. "Because my mother's getting old, and I want to be able to have her over on the weekends."

"How old is she?" I asked.

"Ninety-five" was the reply. "She likes to be able to visit me on weekends."

I had thought I was speaking to *the* senior citizen, and here there were two generations of seniors, a phenomenon that is becoming more and more common toward the end of this century. Nevertheless, Mrs. Dolzani did get away to Las Vegas, passing over the snow-covered Rockies in October, having a good look at the Grand Canyon, and then landing to be bussed into town to the Dunes.

"What do you get out of traveling?" I asked Dolzani. She thought for a second. "It's really like medicine—yes, it's like medicine. When you're traveling you forget all your problems. Then when you come home you're okay—until you get that itchy feeling again. And you meet so many nice people, you know. I'm never afraid to travel alone now. You know you always meet somebody, and people are so nice."

IF, AS COWPER said, variety is the spice that gives life all its flavor, then let me introduce you to a lady whose life contains about as much flavor as it can hold. Skin diving, blacksmithing, and sailing are among the activities she has practiced since she turned sixty.

For about ten years, I used to sail a small cabin sloop out of a port on the East Coast. I had a little dinghy for getting from the town dock out to the boat, and often, while getting the oars out, I would encounter a lady named Barbara, working around the dock. She had curly gray hair and wind-burned cheeks and was clearly no stranger to the

Variety

sea. Her own twenty-six-foot sloop was moored nearby, and I often saw her coiling rope, handling anchors, and doing other mariner-like chores. We would chat about the weather, and I thought about how nice it was that this middle-aged (elderly?) lady got out of doors and kept active. It was a friendly but superficial relationship.

Then, about three years ago, I stopped sailing from that harbor. I didn't see her again until a couple of weeks ago. I was watching some television show when a segment came on depicting the joys of windsurfing. I clicked off the sound and thought about the stupidity of the young today who think that bouncing around on waves close to shore on one of those things was sailing. That was a natural reaction for someone like me who knew perfectly well he could never master the contraption. I had just begun watching the antics on the screen when a familiar face flashed across riding a sailboard with all the skill and aplomb of a young brown-skinned boy at Waikiki. It was Barbara. Dressed in short, frayed blue jean cutoffs and a striped T-shirt, she was leaning back, balancing the force of the wind on the sail, and quite in command of the situation. For a moment she looked at the camera, flashed a smile of victory, and returned her attention to riding her briny broncho.

To say that I was amazed would be an understatement. I had always been absolutely certain that nobody over twenty-six could even attempt windsurfing. I went down to the town dock the next day, where I didn't find Barbara, but where somebody told me that she had become the local agent for windsurfers. For the first time I learned her last name, Coburn, and a phone number where I could reach her. We made an appointment, and a few days later, I drove into her driveway. Outside of the garage there were four cars, one of which appeared in running order. Through the open garage door I saw a moped, a motorcycle, and ten or more stacked sailboards; sails and masts were piled nearby. The various cars appeared to have been left where they died, with a new one added and operational as needed. Although the grass was knee-high, there was nothing slovenly about the appearance of the place; it just looked as though the owner's priorities were elsewhere—in fact, at the harbor and out on salt water.

LIFE BEGINS AT SIXTY

Barbara greeted me warmly at the door, led me into a living room that looked truly lived in, and offered me cider, which I accepted. "Sit down, if you can find a place," she invited, clearing books off a chair. Every flat surface was piled with books and various nautical objects. The walls were solid with nautical paintings, square riggers, ships in fierce storms, Spanish galleons at night; and time, in this maritime museum, was marked every quarter hour by the sounding of ships' bells from several ships' clocks. For me, a lover of everything related to the sea, the room was a treasure, speaking in every corner of its owner's love of the sea. When we settled down to talk, I had to ask Barbara her age; sixty-two, she said. Since I maintain that the sixties are the childhood of senior citizenship, Barbara is indeed a child of that period. And her wide-eyed curiosity and bubbling enthusiasm about a multitude of activities proved me right.

I mentioned having seen her windsurfing on television and asked her how she got involved in the sport. It was a few years ago and she was working at the boatyard. While bicycling past a nearby harbor she saw her first sailboard being handled by young local sailors. Her eyes lit up as she told me, "I watched them bouncing over the waves, and right away, I said, 'Boy, that's for me.' I took a couple of lessons, and then I knew I wanted a board. A couple of more lessons and I bought a boat. The next Labor Day I took it up to Buzzards Bay where my brother and I have a house. That was a rough place to learn, what with the waves and winds of twenty knots, gusting up to thirty. I was having a tough time controlling the board, and that's when I started to read about it and found—'Oh, this is what I should be doing.' That was the start, and the next summer I got much better. Then I sold a couple, and we started a little fleet of them.

"In Europe," Barbara continued, "they took over like wildfire. The reaction there was, 'Well, that looks like a lot of fun...I want to try it.' The reaction in this country was, 'Oh, that looks like a lot of work' [pretty close to my reaction, I'm afraid.] So, late that summer, I got started selling them and teaching people. Some boards are easier—you know, more stable, and with a small sail and when it's not too

Variety

wavy—that's the way to start. I got a lot of people windsurfing that way."

After covering the subject of windsurfing, we got to talking generally about sailing in different parts of the world, and Barbara brought up Cooperstown, New York, where I had once raced on the lake at the age of seventeen. After I described my sailing feats to her, she said, "Oh, when I got up there last, I took the courses in blacksmithing at the Farmer's Museum." She certainly didn't look like a blacksmith to me, but I was getting prepared to expect almost anything from this lady. "Well, what else have you done that I wouldn't guess?" I asked.

"Oh, diving, at the boatyard—just in the line of duty—scuba diving, you know, finding moorings, picking up people's wallets for them, outboards that got away from someone, and changing propellers under water. Just recently we had a boat that sank, a twenty-foot inboard-outboard. I dove down and put lines on it. Then, we tied barrels—at low tide—onto it, and then, when the tide came up [six to eight feet in this location] it raised the boat. I dragged it in as far as I could with the skiff and, then, got a line to shore, and we pulled it in with the tractor."

"How much did that cost the people?" I asked.

"Oh we didn't change 'em anything. Later they brought some Bristol Cream over," she laughed. "I change a lot of propellers under water."

All in a day's work for this lady who surely gets more variety into her life than some would want. On the other hand, here she is at sixty-two, trim, muscular, rosy cheeked, and with eyes as clear as the water in the Caribbean. For me Barbara's eyes are her outstanding feature. With crinkled skin at the edges as have most airplane pilots and sailors (perhaps from always looking at the horizon in bright light), they are eyes with a certain innocence—expectant, always looking for something new. I'm certain that Barbara has no fears for the present and few for the future as she meets life head on with all the vitality and expectancy of a child. Well, didn't I say that the sixties are the childhood of the older years?

LIFE BEGINS AT SIXTY

Walking through the entrance hall, as I prepared to leave, Barbara picked up something off a table. "Here's something new," she said as she held out a pair of knee pads. "These have hard plastic caps for better protection."

"Protection from what?" I asked.

"Well, I've rigged up a six-foot skateboard," she described it, "with wheels front and back. Now I'm trying to rig a mast and sail on it. I think it'll go great in a parking lot—and the best will be on ice. But I wouldn't try it without a helmet."

I'm not going to try it *with* a helmet. But I'm darned sure I'll try windsurfing next summer. And I'm going to try one other experience I've always wanted to have—gliding in a sailplane. I put in a lot of hours flying powered aircraft during World War II, but I've always had a yearning to see what the silent flight of gliding would be like. So there, Barbara's story has already worked a good effect on me. What about you?

9

Hanging in There

The good are better made by ill,
As odors crushed are sweeter still.
— Samuel Rogers

Have you ever read about someone being legally blind and wondered just what it meant? Well Robert Thompson, who is seventy-six years old, has been legally blind for a year. Thompson's blindness, the result of glaucoma, struck particularly hard since he is an unusually active person. He is chairman of the board of trustees of his church; on the advisory council of a local community college; member of the council for the aged at a nearby university; member of the retired teachers association, and a member of the board of management of the YMCA. And eight years ago, Thompson retired from the position of assistant principal of a large metropolitan high school. I asked him how he handled the onset of blindness at this point in his life. "Well," he said, "I treat it something like the story of the man who complained because he had no shoes—until he came across a man who had no feet. Of course, I've felt frustrated and impatient—I hate to ask people to drive me—but I've noticed that my other senses have started to improve, and not just senses. Strangely, my memory has become much sharper. It was always good, but now, it is exceptional."

This runs counter to the old myth that people's memories fail as they age and agrees with new findings that mental abilities continue to improve, perhaps at a more modest rate, even into old age. In Thompson's case, blindness may well have acted as a spur to sharpening his recall. "You see, I believe that everything happens for a reason. I may not have the answer right now, but that makes it easier for me to accept it. I'm not a religious fanatic, but I believe that in His plan there is a reason."

"I've had a good life and a full life up to now," said Thompson, "and I don't intend to let it end there." He reminisced for a few moments. He had spent World War II in the army in the South Pacific, fighting his way from Australia up that long chain of islands toward Japan. His thirty-five years in the public school system had been most rewarding. "Regardless of what people say today," he observed, "the great majority of kids are still mighty good. Of course, there's a percentage of really rotten apples, but most of the trouble with them is we adults. They need and want guidance and discipline." He grinned, "I often have former students come up to me in the street and ask if I still have that 'board' of education! It wasn't a board, really. It was a little paddle I kept in my desk. But it sure did some educating in its time." He thought a moment. "The trouble is, parents substitute sentimentality for love."

There he hit one of my most sensitive nerves about human relations today. We're up to our ears in sentimentality in the movies, television, politics, and on and on. Everybody is going around saying how much they love each other, when it's what you do that counts. Enough of that or I'll bore you stiff.

The point here is that Bob Thompson's life exemplifies the title of this chapter. Though mostly blind and unable to read, he intends to hang right in there and go on making his contribution. He is continuing as chairman of the board of trustees of his church and on the advisory council of the community college; he meets regularly with even greater effectiveness on the university council for the aged; he'll go to the next meeting of the retired teachers association, "if I can get a ride"; and although he is an emeritus member of the management board of the YMCA, he's going to give them the benefit of his thoughts as long as they want them. Thompson has a lot of guts.

Hanging in There

Maybe the fact that he is black and had plenty of obstacles to overcome starting out helps.

"Why do you want to go on doing all these things?" I asked him. "I'm getting on in age, that's true," he said, "but I still don't want to sit around and do nothing. It's an outlet for one thing, and I think I can do some good here and there. I liked to do them all, and then," he paused, "I guess there's always the ego. You know I've got a little ego."

Thank God he's got a little ego.

LET'S REVISIT SOMEONE who makes the affirmative statement "I am" as strongly as anyone I've ever come across. Ruby Hemenway, who writes a weekly newspaper column, who is approaching 101 years of age, and who has been having trouble with her eyes. She has had two operations, if you remember, and her doctor had told her he hoped she would be able to see as well as when she was fifty. I talked to her yesterday. Unfortunately, her eyesight has not improved. She can see just well enough—"if I lean down close to the paper"—to continue writing her weekly columns. She is hopeful that her sight will improve sometime in the future, but for the moment, she also is probably legally blind. Yet she goes right on with her life, brushing aside the disability like a nuisance fly. How does she handle the inevitable problems of daily life? I talked to the editor who handles Hemenway's columns at the *Greenfield Recorder*, Irmarie Jones.

"She's on automatic pilot right now," her editor said. "She's turning them out—it's incredible since she can barely see—but she's worried about having enough columns on hand, so I think we're four or five ahead right now." I asked Irmarie Jones about how she manages at home. "Well, she pretty well takes care of herself," she said. "She has a home health aide once a day for about half an hour. The aide does the lunch dishes and her laundry once a week. But every morning Ruby gets herself up. She takes her bath and dresses herself and makes her own bed. Then, she has 'meals on wheels' five days a week. They wanted to bring her lunch seven days a week, but she wouldn't have it. The health aide leaves her something to warm up for breakfast, but otherwise, she's on her own." Jones said that for long distances Ruby does use a walker, but around the house she just moves around by feeling things.

"Here's an example of how she lives," Jones continued. "She went out about two weeks ago—the Greenfield Women's Club had invited her to speak. They picked her up—it was about a five-mile drive—and when she got there, she spoke sitting down . . . for perhaps forty-five minutes. When it was over, she said, 'I hope I told them everything they wanted to know,' still wondering a little why they wanted to hear her at all. Well, they were enthralled," Jones said, "and her voice, you know, is so clear and strong."

The fact that she did accept the invitation and did go out and speak to the club is Hemenway's way of "hanging in there." She won't let go of life. Instead she continues, with everything she does every day, to make herself a participant in life.

ALZHEIMER'S DISEASE. HERE'S a phrase that strikes fear into the hearts of many, including me. Loss of a limb, loss of sight, loss of hearing, all these would be hard to bear. But when I think of Alzheimer's, I see myself losing the ability to interpret—to make sense of whatever comes into my brain—losing contact with the people I love, and even those I don't love; and I realize I don't want to lose contact with anyone. I see myself floating in total disorientation, like a spacewalker, turning slowly forever in black space with no mother ship to return to. What follows is no effort to diminish the realities of Alzheimer's, but rather, an attempt to meet it and get to know it for what it really is.

Ernest Systrom was born in 1896 and grew up in Wellesley, Massachusetts. His parents could afford a good education for him, and he entered Harvard during World War I only to be interrupted by the entry of the United States into the conflict. He attended officer training school and was close to being sent to France when the war came to an end. Returning to Harvard, he graduated with the class of 1922 with an engineering degree, worked for someone else for a couple of years, and then, started his own venture, the Systrom Company,

Hanging in There

which he headed until his retirement fifty years later at the age of seventy-eight. I first met "Ernie" Systrom when he was eighty-eight, three years after he had been diagnosed as having Alzheimer's disease. He knew I was writing a book about older people and had left word at the office of the senior center where he goes five days a week that I would find him in the gym exercising. When I looked through the glass window in the door, I saw some fourteen seniors, seated in chairs arranged in a semicircle, doing leg exercises led by a forty-year-old physical therapist. I later learned that their ages ranged from sixty-four to ninety-two, and that all of this group were keenly interested in keeping their physical condition sharp. The exercises the therapist led them in were far from the gyrations we see in the health clubs on television. Seated, they slowly raised one leg from rest to the horizontal in front of themselves, held it to a count of five, then, slowly lowered the leg. Same with the other leg. Then, standing behind the chair and holding onto it for balance, they bent knees slowly to a half squat. Obviously, this was not the jogger, sit-up, push-up crowd. The ninety-two-year-old took part as enthusiastically as the rest. But every one of the fourteen was keenly interested in keeping the body supple and ready to respond to the wishes of the mind.

Ernie Systrom stood next to the ninety-two-year-old. He was nattily dressed in slacks, tweed jacket, blue shirt, and striped tie and looked as though he could have just walked out of an ad agency meeting on Madison Avenue. His face was clear, lightly lined, and showing a healthy glow from the mild exercise. His eyes were blue, clear as the summer sky, and his hair, while thin, still showed a faint brown. Seeing me in the door (we had met earlier), he waved me in, and I joined in the activities until the conclusion fifteen minutes later. I noticed that when the participants walked around to the front of their chairs to sit down again, Systrom helped his neighbor (who seemed to have a bad knee) get into his chair. Later, Ernie explained to me, "I have to watch out for him. You know he's ninety-two years old." That comment pretty well sums up the kindly nature of this man.

Although Systrom's company was highly successful and must have taken a good deal of his time throughout his life, his real love, as he

LIFE BEGINS AT SIXTY

tells it now, was always golf. For fifty years he was a member of the Woodland Golf Club in Auburndale, Massachusetts. He was twice president and twice champion of the club and was good enough to have played with Bobby Jones and Walter Hagen. However, he was forced to give up golf two years ago because of arthritis in his hands.

But Ernie determined that he was not through with golf. Along with his other exercises, he has concentrated especially on the hands. Many times a day, he flexes those fingers, working them separately and then opposing each other. Finger by finger, he has brought them back to normal function, until he proudly demonstrated to me the little finger of his left hand. "This was my final conquest," he announced proudly, crooking the last holdout and straightening it several times. I have clear evidence, through his bone-crushing handshake, that this man will surely wield a golf club again. Spring is now a few months away, and a nine-hole town golf course is available. Systrom has been invited to use the course without charge.

I've been emphasizing the physical aspect of Systrom's life because I am convinced after what I've seen that the physical and mental aspects of any person work on and for each other. I know from firsthand experience how the physical affects the mental with me. Normally, I'm a pretty cheerful person. But, like everybody, I occasionally suffer from bouts of depression. I found the cure for me strictly by chance many years ago, and that cure is strenuous physical activity. It can be something like splitting logs for the fireplace, sawing logs (which I hate), raking leaves, or digging holes and planting a bunch of tulips or daffodils for next year. There are two requirements, I think—it must be at least moderately heavy work, and it should be out of doors.

Here we have been talking about a man who has had Alzheimer's disease for three years. I wouldn't be surprised if you'd forgotten that fact as I described his life. Although some very interesting research that seems to point toward meaningful alleviation of the disease has been going on at Dartmouth Medical School, it is still an intellectually crippling disease. I haven't mentioned the fact that Systrom was constantly forgetting my first name—calling me Jim instead of Bill—and yet he was aware of the fact that he was making a mistake and often asked what my name really was. Our several different interviews were a little like starting all over again; though once we got going, he would then recall the purpose of our talks and continue in a helpful way. Although he may have forgotten some things, there was nothing wrong with his business common sense. We were talking about money, although I don't delve into that aspect of anyone's life, and it was clear that Ernie had provided for himself realistically. He told me how a friend had just tried to get him to make an investment "that would pay off handsomely in ten to fifteen years." "What kind of foolishness is that," he chuckled, "telling someone who's eighty-eight about making a lot of money in fifteen years?"

What lies ahead for eighty-eight-year-old Ernie Systrom? We don't know any more than we know what awaits me next week, or a three-day-old baby going home from the hospital with its mother today. To be driving off the first tee on the local golf course early next spring is what Systrom works toward. And to have brought strength and agility back to those arthritic hands is his current accomplishment. Who knows what he can accomplish with a brain that struggles daily against the assault of Alzheimer's disease? And who knows what the work at Dartmouth Medical School, or elsewhere, will result in? What we do know is that, today, Ernie lives, jokes with his friends, keeps up his exercises, and takes care of his ninety-two-year-old friend. Living just now with his daughter, he keeps in close touch with his two sons and, among his grandchildren, with one who is a physician. Isn't that all worth getting up for in the morning?

THE LITTLE GIRL was four and one-half years old when she inadvertantly pushed a small stick into one eye. But that small accident was to change her life entirely. Shortly after that, she completely lost the sight of that eye and the doctor told her parents that it should be removed because it might affect the functioning of the remaining eye. They decided not to have the eye removed because of the effect it would have on her looks. But as months passed the validity of the doctor's prognosis became apparent. By the time she was six years old, Lorraine Berger was totally blind. Now, eighty-four years later, she remembers the events surrounding her loss of sight as clearly as she does the stars in the sky of 1901.

I mention the sky particularly because this cheerful ninety-year-old, who moved into a convalescent home only three years ago, told me with vivid detail how her mother and sister helped her to store up memories before she lost her sight at the age of six. "My mother and oldest sister used to keep showing me the color of things—of roses, the green of the grass, and the blue of the sky. I especially remember one night when my sister took me out—it was a bright starry night, and we spent a long time just looking at the moon and those twinkling stars and talking about what they might mean and how beautiful it all was. I don't think I really knew exactly why she was doing it at the time. Later, of course, we talked about it, and she told me how she had been trying to make memories for me for when I would never be able to see those things again. And do you know, I can still see that sky as though it had been last night."

Ms. Berger (pronounced "Berzher" in the French style) was sitting alertly in her armchair as she told me about the things she saw in 1901. She is a small lady, soigné in every sense of the word; and when she talked to me, she looked straight at me. It is somewhat disconcerting to be stared at by a person you know cannot see.

This lady retired from regular work at the age of seventy-two, which gives you some idea of the kind of person we're dealing with. She had attended a school for the blind until the eighth grade. "Then, well," she explained, "I educated myself pretty well. I always loved to read, and I certainly did an awful lot of reading." The reading, of course, was in braille. She had a braille watch on the table by her chair; and when I noticed a typewriter across the room, yes, that was braille, too.

"I really started working," Ms. Berger relates, "when I heard about all those people who had lost their sight *after* they had grown up. Most of them were so shocked by it that they thought they weren't going to be able to keep house or shop or really do anything. Then I heard about the state board of education's services for the blind. Right away I thought 'that's for me,' I could help blind people, and I could

Hanging in There

earn my own living. It was a regular job, and I did it for forty-four years. I was able to help others as well as help myself."

"But wasn't it difficult teaching others when you were unable to see, too?" I asked.

"You know, I think it helped," she said. "I'd listen to their story first. Then gradually I'd try to get them started on cleaning and cooking. And one of the most important things is that I taught them braille. You see the greatest problem was that they thought life was over. But I knew better."

She certainly did. Ms. Berger lived alone in her own house until she was eighty-seven years old. When she finally entered the convalescent home, she immediately looked around for something to do—and found it. The director of the home told me with satisfaction how she had done wonders in teaching the staff better techniques and attitudes for coping with blind patients when they were admitted. Ms. Berger "listens" to her television set, follows the fortunes "of my Mets" avidly, keeps up her correspondence, and reads her braille edition of *The New York Times* every week. I finally left her room with the conviction that here was a lady who wasn't just "hanging in there" but who was living a fuller life than many who see a great deal but comprehend less.

"THERE ISN'T GOING to be any wheelchair," those are the words that could serve as the theme of the recent life of Dr. Gilbert Leib, of Waterford, Connecticut. Leib is in his middle fifties but his responses to the problems of life are so typical of those that a healthy, adaptive past-sixty-year-old ought to make that I don't feel guilty at including him here. Coming home from the hospital after several weeks and the amputation of his left leg at the knee, Dr. Leib had asked his wife where the wheelchair was. Her reply characterized the spirit with which they both approached the situation of living with a single leg. "I had been using the wheelchair in the hospital," Dr. Leib said. "Then, after I left, I just didn't think. Of course, I still go into the hospital daily—I have to put in so many hours of postgraduate work.

LIFE BEGINS AT SIXTY

But I'm getting better day by day." Leib had the amputation a little less than six months ago, but it was the result of twenty years of slow progression of diabetes that finally resulted in circulation problems in the leg. "I'd had one bypass operation on that leg two years ago, and then they wanted to do another that might last for two more years. Strangely, I was ready to accept the amputation, but the doctors at the hospital wanted to try another bypass. Finally, I told them straight out, 'I was willing to try it once, but that's enough.'" And thus, firmly, Leib moved on to the next stage in his life.

He told me he has a policy of knowing when it's time to say "good-bye." And with this he was referring to almost every aspect of life—or death. "I think there is a time when you should just wash your hands and say 'good-bye,'" he said.

"Do you still practice medicine?" I asked.

"Well, I read electrocardiograms at the hospital," he replied. "I just don't practice in the emergency room anymore though—just in nursing homes. And I didn't drive my tractor last summer."

"You mean you have a farm?" I asked.

"No, but there are about three acres of lawn and a pond to take care of."

"You going to try the tractor?"

"Oh yes, next year, I expect I'll be ready to handle it. And I drive the car some now, though I don't drive at night. After all, what do you need a left foot for? I use the right for the accelerator and brake." Leib explained to me that there was a state law requiring notification of the motor vehicle department after a serious hospital stay, but neither he nor his physician had been able to ascertain the name of whom to notify. A state program was started after World War II for retraining returning veterans whose loss of one or more limbs made driving a problem. Leib had secured a booklet from the state on driving for the handicapped, and he read me a short quotation. "Some of our best drivers are the physically handicapped," it stated. Isn't that a fine commentary on the human race, I thought. Life gives them a handicap and they not only rise to the challenge, they rise above it.

Leib's voice has the sharp brilliance that goes with blooming

Hanging in There

health and vigorous mental activity. While he always gave me the time I needed to interview him and made full replies, there was nevertheless a feeling of being eager to get on with whatever was coming next. He continued answering my question about what he does physically now.

"Well, I've spent the last six months learning to walk. Mainly, I'm learning to walk with a cane."

"Is it a tough job?" I asked.

"Mostly stairs and steps," he said. "Hard? Sure it's hard. You have to keep at it. Of course, you keep gaining weight all the time." I started to ask how much weight he had lost after the operation, but then the thought of the missing leg struck me, and I dropped the question fast. "As to what I do," he went on, "Saturday mornings I go down to the church. Cook up a breakfast of potatoes, eggs, sausages, and warm muffins."

"Who for?" I wondered.

"Oh, anybody who wants to come. We ask them to pay two dollars, but if they don't have it, they get breakfast anyway. Then, what we don't give out at the church, we take down to a shelter in the ghetto section of town. We've gotten together, two of our churches, and we're renovating a building—making a shelter to sleep about sixty. I've also gotten involved in the Literacy Volunteers of America. I've been teaching Hispanics in ESL. That's 'English as a second language.' I find that's been a lot of fun. In fact, I guess it's what I enjoy most these days, educating minority groups. You know what I think the biggest problem is? We just don't understand what they don't have." He was talking about what a child learns at home before even going to school —all the language learned from parents, ways of thinking picked up by osmosis from brothers and sisters as well as parents and grandparents. "I enjoy working on the EKG panel, but I guess there's nothing I enjoy as much as working with minority groups. There's nothing else that makes me realize how lucky we are to have come through this world as Americans in the mainstream.

"I go to a lot of parties whenever I can. I have a pretty extensive philatelic library, though I'm beginning to sell off a lot of the stamps now. But," he said, summing it up, "my main pleasure is reading, reading about educating minority groups. And now, I'm on the board of directors of the Literacy Volunteers of America."

Dr. Leib paused thoughtfully for a moment. I think he was wondering whether to make his next comment or not. "You have to watch out though when you go into those neighborhoods where the shelters are," he said, finally. "I remember coming out of the shelter one night. There was a man a little way down the street. When I got to him, I saw that he was about ready to tear me apart."

"I don't know what you mean," I said.

"He wanted money—ten dollars or anything, a watch or whatever. And I couldn't walk very fast. I told him I didn't have anything. I just had my driver's license in my shoe, upside down. He asked, 'Don't you have anything?' I told him, 'I don't even have a hat.' And do you know what he said? he said, 'Oh, hell, I must be in the wrong place.' And he shook his head and walked away."

Gilbert Leib has had an artificial leg fitted since I first spoke to him and seems to be adapting well to its use. How will he shape the years to come? How will he use his skills and experience now? I certainly don't know. But what I believe I know is that he will bring vigor, intelligence, and a high degree of sensitivity to whomever and whatever he works with. Hanging in there? I could never see him doing anything else.

10

The Man Who Did Everything

Too busy with the crowded hour to fear to live or die.
— Emerson

Perhaps the time has come for a change of pace. Until now we have looked at a number of role models in each chapter—people who seem to have handled their lives extremely well in those areas that I think are vital for a long, fully realized and happy life—areas such as retirement, goals, life expectancy, variety, doing good, and so on. Now, instead of a little about many, I want to tell you a lot about one person.

In visualizing this book, I made a decision to steer clear of the lives of famous people who achieved greatness and happiness into their eighties and nineties. Possibly like you, I found myself saying, "Well, if I had his genius, her talent, his money, I'd live to be a happy ninety-five, too!" So the rule has been to stay away from the rich and famous and tell the stories of real people like you and me. Still, there is always the exception that proves the rule. His name is Benjamin Franklin.

LIFE BEGINS AT SIXTY

What follows is the story of those aspects of his life, as it unfolded between the ages of fifty-nine and eighty-four, that exemplify the chapter headings at the beginning of this book. And when you see all those positive qualities illustrated in Franklin's life, I'm going to ask you to relate them to the way you live. When you see Franklin trying to obtain millions of livres from the French king to finance the Revolution in America, think of raising a few hundred or thousand dollars for a good cause in your hometown. When you see him planning European tours to expand his mind, look for a trip you might take to amuse and instruct yourself.

The time was November 1764. The brig, a two-masted sailing ship, rolled slowly in the light wind, some 150 miles to the east of Long Island, at the start of a four-week trip to England. Near the stern, on the starboard side, in the shadow of the great mizzen, an elderly gentleman was leaning far out over the rail. The ship's captain watched him as he slowly paid out a line with a weight on the end. This was the ship's lead, used to determine the depth of the water. But here, beyond the continental shelf, there was no chance of reaching bottom.

"Have you taken any readings yet, Dr. Franklin?" the skipper asked.

"We may just be on the edge now, sir," the noted scientist replied. He waited a few moments and then pulled the line back in. Just above the lead weight at the end, a thermometer was attached to the line. He read the water temperature and smiled. It had risen three degrees since his reading an hour earlier.

Franklin was now certain that the ship had entered the Gulf Stream. Since his first trip to England at the age of eighteen, he had had great interest in that warm-water river meandering in a salty ocean. His first information had come from a cousin, Captain Timothy Folger, of Nantucket, who gave him some idea of the dimensions and direction of the stream, and true to his unquenchable curiosity, Franklin never failed to grasp any opportunity to enlarge his knowledge of the phenomenon. He was the first scientist to study and report on this anomaly in the North Atlantic.

The Man Who Did Everything

The more I learned about Franklin, the more I became convinced that a lively curiosity was his major character trait. It sometimes led him into danger, but I think the knowledge gained was greater than the risks he took. After all, Franklin was no amateur scientist. His earlier work with electricity, the first lead-plate electric battery, lightning rods, the Franklin stove (still unsurpassed for economical heating), the first water tank for testing ship's hulls, and endless scientific conclusions drawn from firsthand observation had already earned him membership in the Royal Society of England, and a degree of Doctor of Civil Law from Oxford University.

Yet now, in his fifty-ninth year, Franklin was not traveling to England as a scientist but, rather, as something close to a diplomat. He had been chosen by the Pennsylvania General Assembly to carry a petition to King George III. He had represented the colony of Pennsylvania earlier in a stay of five years in England, attempting to lessen the grip of the Penn family on its colony in the New World. Now friction between Great Britain and its American colonies was growing steadily and producing more and more heat. As early as 1751, Franklin had voiced his own first warning to the mother country when he wrote on Britain's practice of deporting convicted criminals to the American colonies. Writing as "Americanus," he noted what the British called the "improvement and well peopling of America" and suggested that this motherly concern surely deserved some kind of like repayment. He noted that "in some of the uninhabited parts of these provinces there are numbers of venomous reptiles we call rattlesnakes, felons convict from the beginning of the world." Franklin's observation was that these creatures might "possibly change their natures if they were to change their climate," and so he suggested that "some thousands might be collected annually and transported to Britain." There he suggested that they could be "carefully distributed in St. James Park, in the Spring Gardens and other places of pleasure about London; in the gardens of all the nobility and gentry thoughout the nation; but particularly in the gardens of the prime ministers, the lords of trade, and members of Parliament, for to them we are most particularly obliged."

LIFE BEGINS AT SIXTY

He further suggested that Britain would have the best of the bargain because the "rattlesnake gives warning . . . which the convict does not." Yet fourteen years later, measuring the temperature of the Gulf Stream from a packet bound for England, Franklin's goal was still the preservation of the empire.

When he arrived at the Isle of Wight on December 9, 1764, Franklin's objective was to see that the Penn family was no longer allowed to own and rule the province of Pennsylvania but, rather, be forced to sell it to the king so that it would be administered like the other colonies. The descendants of William Penn, particularly a grandson, Thomas Penn, insisted on ruling the colony in a far more dictatorial and high-handed manner than the king applied to the other colonies. Pennsylvania was a proprietary grant from the crown, and this was what Franklin had been sent to change.

When he reached London, Franklin went straight to the home of Margaret Stevenson, where he had rented rooms on an earlier trip. The lodgings were exceedingly comfortable, and I gather that Franklin enjoyed a warm relationship with Mrs. Stevenson—to say the least. Earlier in a letter, "Advice to a Young Man on the Choice of a Mistress," after stating that marriage was the proper remedy for sexual desires, he went on to say: "In all your amours you should prefer old women to young ones." He listed all his sound reasons for the advice and wound up with "And, lastly, they are so grateful." I suspect Franklin was probably following his own advice. The only direct evidence I have of this is a sketch by the painter, Charles Wilson Peale, who had arrived unannounced at the Stevenson house and found Franklin seated with an attractive woman on his knee. Peale's sketch shows the couple engaged in what was then delicately known as dalliance. To be a little more specific, it is a scene that would not be permitted on your television screen today—well, unless you subscribed to a certain cable network.

Events moved very slowly in those times. It could easily require three months for a message to make the round trip to America and back. The king and nobles took their long summers away from work, and any personal business of these nobles and ministers took prece-

The Man Who Did Everything

dence over government affairs, particularly, those of the American colonies. And so, however anxious he was to make progress, Franklin too found plenty of leisure time.

In spite of his earlier five-year stint representing the Pennsylvania General Assembly, Franklin was still far better known in England and Europe as a scientist. And his stature was not based only on his work with electricity, though that was the best known. He observed, and experimented on, everything that came under his eye. Early in his teens, Franklin, always a great swimmer, made some paddles with holes for his thumbs, which he found greatly increased his swimming speed. He also developed a kind of large sandal to act as flippers on his feet. An avid kite flyer, he one day decided to combine kite flying with swimming. After getting the kite aloft, he attached a stick to the line for a handle and, floating on his back, allowed himself to be pulled across a lake—first arranging for another boy to carry his clothes to the other side. I find the picture of Franklin sailing feet first across the lake unforgettable. The only difficulty was that if he moved too fast the kite would naturally descend. He solved this problem by braking with his feet in the water. Interestingly, he says he did this only once. I guess he saw no future in the method of transportation.

The popular picture of Franklin and his kite is that of flying the kite in a thunderstorm, with a key on the string, and hoping it would be struck by lightning. In fact, Franklin hoped for no such thing; he probably knew such a result would be fatal. Earlier he had already invented and made an electric storage battery and nearly killed himself using it to electrocute a turkey before "roasting it by the electrical jack." He had mistakenly grabbed the wrong pole in one hand. There was a great flash, a crack like a pistol, and Franklin fell unconscious to the ground.

Nobody knew at the time whether lightning was a form of electricity or not; and to resolve this was Franklin's purpose in flying the kite. With the help of his son, William, he raised the kite on a stormy day and waited for a dark thundercloud. The first one caused no visible effect. Soon, however, Franklin observed the hairs of the string beginning to stand erect and separate from each other. When he touched the key he saw and felt small electric sparks. Later, when the rain wet the string, a good deal more electric fire was seen, and Franklin now knew for sure that lightning and electricity were one and the same thing. The useful outcome of the experiment was the first lightning rod. Another result was a further honor for Franklin. At the age of sixty-six, he was chosen Associé Etrangère (foreign member) of the Royal Academy in Paris, a sign of great respect from the first academy in the world. There were only seven other such members.

Almost nothing escaped Franklin's inquiring eye. A few years later, while traveling in Holland, he observed the canal boats. He asked about their speed and was told that they traveled faster when the water in the canal was deep and more slowly when it became shallow. "Why?" the true scientist immediately asked himself. He reasoned that the canal boat "must in every boat's length of her course move out of her way a body of water equal in bulk to the room her bottom took up in the water." He then concluded that this water had to go to the sides and under the boat. But when shallow water prevented it from going under, it would pile up against the sides and slow the boat.

He built a wooden tank fourteen feet long, which he filled with water, and a small boat that could be pulled through it. From the bow of the boat, he ran a small thread along the surface of the water and over a smoothly turning brass pulley at the end. For a weight he attached a shilling to the thread. Then, placing the boat at one end, he allowed the weight to pull it the length of the trough. Counting carefully, he timed the boat's progress at different water depths. In one and one-half inches of water, it took a count of 101 to travel the fourteen feet; and in four and one-half inches of water, the boat made the trip in a count of only seventy-nine. Franklin had proved his point, and in so doing, invented the hull testing tank, reinvented today, particularly, for use in designing racing hulls for ships such as the America's Cup contenders. He then left it to the Dutch to decide whether the expense of deepening their canals would be worth the increased speed of travel.

As 1765 wore on, news came from the colonies of rioting against the Stamp Act. When the hated stamps actually arrived in the colonies, they were rarely used, and business went on as usual without them. Franklin was surprised at the violent reaction against the stamps, although he clearly understood and backed the resistance to the idea of the colonists being taxed by a body in which they had no representation. For months Franklin worked quietly to encourage opposition to the act. He wrote anonymous letters to newspapers, used his wit and incisive logic to influence the influentials, and finally, published in the *London Chronicle* his own statement on the overall American position. With all these activities, he was getting ready for an extraordinarily important event: the appearance of the most important American in Europe (himself) as a witness before the House of Commons.

Testifying before the House of Commons, he drew attention away from the dangerous distinction between internal and external taxes by making what was really a veiled threat: we don't need your exports. And, also, he made the threat crystal clear as to the crippling blow this would be to English manufacturers. Later, he boasted privately in a letter to his wife, Deborah: "Had the trade between the two countries ceased it was a comfort to me to recollect that I had once been clothed from head to foot in woolen and linen of my wife's manufacture... I told Parliament that it was my opinion, before the old clothes of the Americans wore out they might have new ones of their own making. And indeed if they all had as many clothes as your old man has, that would not be very unlikely, for I think you and George reckoned when I was last at home at least twenty pair of old breeches." In the same letter after the repeal of the act, he mentioned some gifts he was sending Deborah and his daughter, Sally. "Joking apart, I have sent you a fine piece of Pompadour satin, fourteen yards, cost 11 shillings a yard; a silk negligee and brocaded lutestring [a glossy silk cloth] for my dear Sally, with two dozen gloves, four bottles of lavender water."

After the Stamp Act was repealed, relations between Britain and the colonies quieted. Franklin was cheered as a hero—on both sides of the Atlantic.

Shortly after this victory, Franklin asked the Pennsylvania General Assembly to let him return to America. Instead they appointed him representative for another year; and later, he was appointed agent for Georgia, New Jersey, and finally, in 1770, Massachusetts. In effect, he was now playing a role very close to that of ambassador for America in England although such a function never existed on any table of organization. The salaries for his various jobs amounted to fifteen hundred pounds annually—though they were often paid late—and these, together with other income as owner of printing operations and deputy postmaster general, made him a comparatively rich man and well able to maintain comfortable establishments in both Philadelphia and London. At the same time, a false calm in relations between Britain and America offered Franklin the leisure to pursue his loves of science, travel, and the company of attractive women.

Nobody was better able to get more out of travel than Benjamin Franklin. He now journeyed a great deal through Ireland, Scotland, Holland, Germany, and France. And he took the opportunity of indulging his talent for writing elaborate hoaxes—often for serious ends, but mostly for his own amusement. While still young he had once pointed out, after rationalizing the eating of fish since they also eat one another, what a convenient thing it was to be rational. "So convenient a thing it is to be a reasonable creature, since it enables one to find or make a reason for anything one has a mind to do." In a moment of leisure that resulted from a minor illness, Franklin wrote for an English newspaper under the pseudonym, "A Traveller," a spoof about plans for cod and whale fisheries in the Great Lakes. "Ignorant people may object," he wrote, "that the upper lakes are fresh and that cod and whale are salt water fish. But let them know, Sir, that cod, like other fish when attacked by their enemies fly into any water where they can be safest; that the whales, when they have a mind to eat cod, pursue them wherever they flee; and that the grand leap of the whale in that chase up the Falls of Niagara is esteemed by all who have seen it, as one of the finest spectacles in nature." Americans may have been considered yokels in Britain, but one of them had a lot of Englishmen imagining this fantastic sight.

Franklin was irrepressible, as a single sly sentence he slipped into an otherwise serious letter to Polly Stevenson, the daughter of his land-

The Man Who Did Everything

lady, shows. The letter was a reply to one of hers containing questions about science and nature and dealt with insects, the silkworm, bees, and so on. In the middle of a discourse on their usefulness, appears this dry observation: "The usefulness of the cantharides, or Spanish flies, in medicine is known to all, and thousands owe their lives to that knowledge." Whether he expected Polly to "get" the outrageous comment, we can't be sure, but it is an indication of Franklin's inability to refrain from humor when an opportunity presented itself.

More often, he aimed his satire at serious goals. In 1771, when he was sixty-five and a full five years before the signing of the Declaration of Independence, he wrote a stinging satire about how the British treated the American colonies. Called *Rules by Which a Great Empire Can Be Reduced to a Small One*, it was fictitiously represented as advice to the new ministers to the British Crown. It was really addressed to the earl of Hillsborough, with whom he had feuded since Hillsborough had taken over as manager of colonial affairs. "You are to consider," Franklin advised, "that a great empire, like a great cake, is most easily diminished at the edges." He suggested the minister begin at the remotest provinces and, later, go about losing the nearer ones. And he added that provinces should never be made a part of the mother country. In dealing with the colonies, he suggested, "Suppose them always inclined to revolt, and treat them accordingly. By this means, like the husband who uses his wife ill from suspicion, you may in time convert your suspicions into realities."

Another rule he recommended was "Convert the brave, honest officers of your navy into pimping tide-waiters and colony officers of the customs. And to chase smugglers," he advised, "scour with armed boats every bay, creek, harbor, cove . . . throughout the coast of your colonies. Then let these boats' crews land upon every farm in their way, rob the orchards, steal the pigs and poultry, and insult the inhabitants. If the injured and exasperated farmers should attack the offenders, drub them and burn their boats, you are to call this high treason and rebellion . . . and threaten to carry off all the offenders three thousand miles to be hanged, drawn and quartered. Oh, this will work admirably."

LIFE BEGINS AT SIXTY

A useful deception that he carried out unblushingly over his own name had to do with the famous Baron von Steuben, who later, under General Washington, whipped the amateur American soldiers into an efficient fighting machine in a matter of months. Steuben, who came to Franklin as an unemployed former captain who had served under Frederick the Great, was looking for a job. As a mere captain, he would hardly have received the assignments he did under Washington. But Franklin, knowing of his service on the Prussian general staff and of his high reputation, promoted the German to the rank of "Lieutenant General in the King of Prussia's service" in his letter of recommendation.

Franklin's English stay ended in 1775 when he returned to Philadelphia on the death of his wife. On his return he was immediately appointed by the Pennsylvania General Assembly as deputy to the Second Continental Congress. Now, in his seventieth year, Franklin might well have retired. I can't readily think of many men of that age who engage in revolutions and risk death by hanging for treason. Instead he busied himself furiously for the next year in preparing defenses for America. He first thought of the scheme of floating large log booms in rivers and positioning iron posts and logs to prevent British ships from sailing up to cities such as Philadelphia. He also, at the request of the committee on safety, designed a pike that American soldiers, short of muskets and having no bayonets, could use to withstand the British bayonet charge. During 1775 and 1776, he was busy in every quarter. As a former official of the Royal Post Office, he was now appointed postmaster general and the American Postal System descends almost uninterrupted from the way he organized it for the Continental Congress.

In June 1776, Jefferson, John Adams, and Franklin were the major contributors to a declaration prepared for publication to the world. Jefferson prepared the first draft and showed it to the other two. Franklin's changes, which were few and short, were very much to the point. Where Jefferson had written, "We hold these truths to be sacred and undeniable," Franklin's handwriting changes the last three words to the shorter and stronger "self-evident." That and other changes evidence Franklin's penetrating logic and his ability to hit the bull's-eye, rather than scatter his verbal shots. He also changed Jefferson's "reduce them to arbitrary power" to "reduce them under absolute despotism"—again, stronger language. A true writer, Jefferson remarked later, "I was not insensible to these mutilations." Here is a fleeting glance at the humanness of the Founding Fathers. I can easily visualize Jefferson wincing as Franklin's pen scratched. But I also admire the willingness to sacrifice self for the common good.

On July 4, the document was agreed to by the Congress. The first to sign was John Hancock, as president of the group. He is supposed to have said something like, "There must be unanimity—we must all hang together." At which Franklin supposedly remarked, "Yes, we must all hang together, or assuredly we shall all hang separately."

And the following autumn, Franklin risked hanging in a very real way when he sailed across a very British ocean on his way to represent the fledgling country in Paris. But prior to this, there had been some unsuccessful efforts to settle the war before it became a major bloodletting. On one such occasion Franklin and John Adams, later the second president of the United States, went to Staten Island to meet Lord Howe at his request. On the way the two Americans stayed at an inn in New Brunswick, where it was so crowded that the two had to share one bed in a tiny room. Franklin was a kind of eighteenth-century "health nut" in that he thought a lot of fresh air was vital to health. He even took "air baths" every morning for which he sat naked in his room with windows open wide for one hour. So this night at the inn, he opened the single window wide. Adams said later, "I, who was an invalid and afraid of the night, shut it close. 'Oh,' says Franklin, 'don't shut the window, we shall be suffocated.' And Franklin opened the window saying, 'Come open the window and I shall convince you. I believe you are not acquainted with my theory about colds.'" So Adams allowed the window open and was honest enough to admit that he fell asleep while Franklin was still explaining his theory. He also remembered that the last words he heard were spoken very sleepily. I think that a fine insight into the personalities of the Founding Fathers—the second president of the United States and

LIFE BEGINS AT SIXTY

Franklin, in bed together arguing whether to open the window or not!

The following October, Franklin set sail for France in an armed sloop, knowing full well that if captured, he would almost certainly be hanged for treason. He was even agreeable to the captain's desire to capture two British merchant ships on the voyage, which they brought into a French port. This was quite a trip for a man within a month of his seventy-first birthday, and it did in fact put Franklin out of action for weeks. He had suffered from gout for some time and was so weak on his arrival that he could hardly stand. But, given time and some comfortable living, he was soon set up in Paris in the role of the first ambassador from the new United States.

At the start, things were extremely difficult. Throughout 1777 there were reports of British victories in America, and the French, who could never afford an alliance with America or war against England under such circumstances, sat quietly on the fence, at least publicly. Franklin's role through this difficult period was to sit imperturbably in Paris, shedding a glow of absolute confidence over all negotiations, and keeping the French undecided until America's fortunes turned. In December 1777, such news finally arrived; General Burgoyne had surrendered his entire army at Saratoga. Franklin's tireless negotiation with the French, although he was surrounded by British spies, finally achieved success in January 1778, when the French king let him know that he was ready to sign a treaty of "amity and commerce" immediately. Franklin's victory here was at least the equal of that won against Burgoyne at Saratoga. While Franklin had originally been one of a commission of three from Congress to France, he received, in February 1779, documents appointing him sole plenipotentiary from America, that is, the new country's first ambassador. Because he still suffered badly from gout it was some time before Franklin was able to present himself at court in his new role. But in March, he says in his autobiography, "I thought myself able to go through the ceremony and accordingly went to court in my new character and had my audience with the king, presented my letter of credence, and was received very graciously."

Franklin's other major function as ambassador was the raising of money in large amounts, without which the Congress and the armies of the new country could not possibly wage war. This was at least as important as his successful efforts to set France against England and, probably, more difficult to accomplish. Nevertheless he was able to wheedle many millions of livres in loans and even outright gifts from the French foreign minister and Louis, himself.

Franklin also carried out many other functions for the American Congress in Europe. He seemed to be a jack-of-all-trades as ambassador. Not only was he a kind of secretary of the treasury on that side of the Atlantic but he also functioned as a secretary of the navy, taking care of the fitting out of privateers that plundered British merchant ships right up to the English ports. He saw that John Paul Jones's ship, the *Bonhomme Richard*, was supplied, and fit for sea, from French ports. The ship, named in honor of Franklin, soon won the first American naval victory, defeating the British naval vessel, *Serapis*, within sight of British shores.

Franklin had moved to Passy, then a Parisian suburb, early in his stay in France, and there he was able to enjoy both rest and the things he loved most in life. Always a printer, he set up his own press in Passy and even cast type in his own foundry. He continued his ever-active interest in the world of science and carried on a fairly elaborate social life among his highly civilized neighbors. And although he was seventy-five in 1781, his custom of outrageous flirtations continued.

Still, he attempted to resign his post that year. Perhaps he felt he could no longer represent America as well as he thought it should be. His letter stated, "I have passed my 75th year and I find that the long and severe fit of gout which I had last winter has shaken me exceedingly and I am yet far from having recovered the bodily strength I before enjoyed." He went on to write, "I have been engaged in public affairs and enjoyed public confidence, in some shape or other, during the long term of 50 years, and honour sufficient to satisfy any reasonable ambition; and I have no other left but that of repose, which I hope the Congress will grant me." Congress, however, promptly refused his request, and he seemed delighted with this outcome.

As Franklin had aged, he had become increasingly nearsighted and found it more than a nuisance to keep changing his "spectacles" from reading to wanting to look up at someone. He mentioned that he could not see clearly across the dinner table without one set, nor see his food without the other. He added that he found it far easier to understand French when he could see clearly the face of the speaker. So Franklin took what to him was the obvious remedy. He had the "glasses cut and a half of each kind associated in the same circle." With such great simplicity and direct response to a clear need were bifocal glasses invented by this extraordinary man!

In Passy, Franklin lived in a wing of a lovely chateau belonging to a family named Chaumont; and he apparently dined with that family the first few months he lived there. But he soon set up his own establishment in his wing, complete with printing press, well-stocked wine cellar, and his own majordomo who ran the place. He entertained fairly elaborately as became any ambassador but was careful not to make a show greater than other ambassadors in Paris.

In 1779, there were more than a thousand bottles of wine in his cellar, including red and white Bordeaux, champagne, and also forty-eight bottles of rum. By 1782, his stock showed a couple of hundred more bottles. Apparently his gout was doomed to fight a losing battle against the wine. Franklin had always enjoyed good drink though he strongly disapproved of excessive consumption. In his youth in Philadelphia, he had written a number of jovial drinking songs and spent his share of time in taverns drinking rum and Madeira. I especially like this song he wrote at that time.

> The antediluvians were all very sober,
> For they had no wine, and they brewed no October;
> All wicked, bad livers, on mischief still thinking,
> For there can't be good living where there is not
>   good drinking.

"October" refers to a British ale brewed in that month, something Franklin surely didn't drink in France.

The Man Who Did Everything

Life in Passy also offered this elderly gentleman another pleasure he valued very highly: the company of beautiful women. Of course his position as ambassador attracted many women to his presence. But, nevertheless, it seems clear that they were also attracted by the personality, humor, gracious manner, and perhaps mostly, the sharp intellect of this unusual man.

He formed strong attachments particularly with two of his noble neighbors, Madame Brillon and Madame Helvetius. John Adams, who came to France for peace negotiations in 1780 as the war wound down after Cornwallis's surrender, said somewhat disapprovingly of Franklin that "at the age of seventy-odd he had neither lost his taste for beauty nor his love for it." Although he was seventy-four at the time, Franklin felt it necessary to explain in a letter to a niece in Boston why it was that he was seen to kiss ladies on their necks. It seemed, he said, that when ladies were presented to him, they expected to be embraced, "that is to have their necks kissed. For as to the kissing of lips or cheeks it is not the mode here; the first is reckoned to be rude, and the other may rub off the paint."

Nevertheless, Mme. Brillon, in her thirties and married to a much older treasury official, certainly enjoyed a relationship with Franklin that had a good deal of spice in it. She had once asked him to be a father to her, but they were hardly father and daughter. She once complained to him in a letter that "people have the audacity to criticize my pleasant habit of sitting on your knee, and yours of always asking me for what I always refuse." Though she vowed to be more discreet, she once played chess with him while she sat in her covered bath. He reports they were so absorbed that it was past eleven when he got home.

While he apparently never succeeded in his attempts at conquest, he nevertheless continued to press his amiable attacks as long as he knew Mme. Brillon. He even used his gout as an arguing point. He once asked her to consider the fact that "when I was a young man and enjoyed more favors from the opposite sex than at present, I never had the gout. If the ladies of Passy had more of that Christian charity which I have so often recommended to you, in vain, I would not have the gout now." Apparently his efforts never achieved success, but Mme. Brillon loved him and continued to correspond with him after his return to Philadelphia and as long as he lived.

Another lady with whom Franklin enjoyed a very warm relationship was Mme. Helvetius, a widow who lived in nearby Auteuil with her two daughters. She conducted her salon in the old style and entertained men like Voltaire and the great economist Turgot and, of course, Benjamin Franklin. Mme. Helvetius was so beautiful that the famous writer Fontenelle, who lived to be one hundred, is said to have paid her the great compliment, "Ah, Madame, if I were only eighty again." Franklin, being only seventy-eight, enjoyed a bantering sexual relationship with her—one that shocked John Adams's wife, Abigail, when she dined with Franklin and Mme. Helvetius in 1784. Mrs. Adams, from chilly New England, noted with asperity that the French woman called the famous American doctor simply "Franklin," that she kissed his cheeks and forehead when she greeted him, and that, at dinner, she often held his hand and even threw her arm around his neck. Perhaps what annoyed Abigail even more was that Mme. Helvetius occasionally rested her arm along the back of John Adams's chair. What had been going on here during the peace negotiations, she must have wondered, before she arrived on the scene.

Franklin's attitude toward the lovely Mme. Helvetius is well typified by his reply when she complained that he had postponed a visit she was waiting for. "Madam," he said gallantly, "I have been waiting until the nights are longer." Franklin made many verbal assaults on the lady's virtue, one of the most charming of which had to do with Mme. Helvetius's departed husband and Franklin's wife who was also presumably in heaven. He described a dream in which he found himself in the Elysian fields and encountered Monsieur Helvetius. They discussed current affairs, and then Franklin asked M. Helvetius why he never mentioned his dear wife whom Franklin admired extravagantly. Helvetius stated that he had a new wife and, at that point in the dream, in walked Deborah Franklin. When Franklin attempted to claim her, he told Mme. Helvetius, she said, "I was a good wife to you for 49 years and four months.... Be content with that. I have formed a new connexion here which will last for eternity." At this point in his dream Franklin related to Mme. Helvetius, "I at once resolved to quit those ungrateful shades, return to this good world, and see again the sun and you. Here I am," he said. "Let us avenge ourselves." As far as we know, they never avenged themselves, and the lady remained true to her departed husband.

Nevertheless, like so many of Franklin's close female friends, Mme. Helvetius remained on warm intimate terms with him as long as he lived. On the way to the ship for his final return to America he wrote, "It seems to me that things are badly arranged in this world, when I see two beings made to be happy with each other obliged to separate." Three years later, he wrote her from Philadelphia with evident longing, "Often in my dreams I have breakfast with you. I sit beside you on one of your hundred sofas, I walk with you in your beautiful garden." She also wrote him, sending things for his daughter plus personal presents from herself and saying that she had always loved him and always would. Even though they would never see each other again in this world, perhaps in the next, "we shall meet again, with all those who loved us, I a husband and you a wife—but I believe you have been a rogue and will find more than one."

Finally, after long negotiations, which had come into Franklin's hands as did most matters, a peace treaty was signed in September 1783. Franklin's comment at that time is worth remembering. "In my opinion there never was a good war or a bad peace." He was seventy-seven years old and had worked long and hard, in poor health and good, first to preserve the empire if possible and, finally, seeing that that end was hopeless, to see America a free and independent nation.

By the time he left on his return to America, Franklin was suffering great pain from a bladder stone, which was to bother him on and off for the rest of his life. He could not stand to ride in a carriage and so had to be carried in a litter rigged between two mules, all the way from Paris to the port of Le Havre. Nevertheless, on crossing to England, he was the only passenger not to get seasick. In the few days before leaving Southampton, he came to enjoy the saltwater baths available nearby. Once, he says, "I went at noon to bathe at St. Martin's salt

LIFE BEGINS AT SIXTY

water bath and, floating on my back, fell asleep and slept near an hour by my watch without sinking or turning . . . water is the easiest bed that can be." Had he discovered the water bed?

As soon as the ship for America got into deep water, Franklin again started taking water temperatures and charting the Gulf Stream. He wrote steadily on the trip, which was his eighth crossing of the Atlantic, making suggestions concerning improved rigging of ships and a device to keep heavy ropes from breaking under sudden tension. He also described what is today known as the "sea anchor," a floating canvas cone that will keep a ship headed into the wind and waves, when it is too deep to use an ordinary anchor. Here, he also made the important suggestion of constructing watertight compartments in ships to avoid sinking.

Arriving in America, Franklin still had many honors and achievements ahead of him. But his health was uneven, and the bladder stone gave him little respite. He was immediately elected to the Pennsylvania General Assembly again and later to the office of president of Pennsylvania. He made many important contributions at the constitutional convention in 1787. He was over eighty years old when he signed the document, along with George Washington and others, but certainly strong enough to be able to make a speech in which he pointed out that the document had some shortcomings. (He was later vindicated when it was thought necessary to add the Bill of Rights.) In spite of that, he urged others to sign it, saying, "Thus I consent, Sir, to this constitution because I expect no better, and I am not sure it is not the best." At this time, Franklin was eighty-one. John Adams was fifty-two; Jefferson, forty-four; and Washington, fifty-five—in fact, a younger generation. Perhaps Franklin should be called "Father of the Founding Fathers."

His last public act, carried out when he had only months to live, was to sign a memorandum to Congress urging the abolition of slavery. In fact, in the last month of his life, Franklin sent an elaborate spoof to the *Federal Gazette,* which described the taking of Christian slaves by Algerine pirates and the justification of the practice by one Sidi Mehemet Ibrahim. It was as precise, clear, and satirically sharp as any of his earlier writings in that vein.

The Man Who Did Everything

His pain was by his own description excruciating, yet Franklin continued to live, in every sense of the word, all of his days. He was surrounded by friends. Polly Hewson, the daughter of his old landlady in London, had come with her children to live in the house in Philadelphia. Jefferson called on him, and he enjoyed the company of his grandchildren. Perhaps the words he might like to have remembered as his last are contained in a letter to Ezra Stiles, president of Yale College.

> You desire to know something of my religion.... Here is my creed. I believe in one God, Creator of the universe. That he governs it by his providence. That he ought to be worshipped. That the most acceptable service we can render to Him is to do good to his other children. That the soul of man is immortal, and will be treated with justice in another life.... These I take to be the fundamental principles of all sound religion, and I regard them as you do in whatever sect I meet them.

Leaving these words, Franklin died a few days later.

11

Sex After Sixty

> It's too good for them, Damme, out of my garden!
> —Louis XV

Reportedly, the unforgettable words above were spoken by Louis XV of France when, while strolling in the gardens of Versailles with his majordomo, he came across a servant girl and her boyfriend making sport in the bushes. "What are they doing?" the astounded king asked his majordomo.

"F------, Sire," the majordomo replied, with admirable precision. Whereupon the king articulated the comment at the top of this page.

Unfortunately, a large number of the young and middle-aged today still take the same attitude toward sex for the grandparent set. To coin a Victorian phrase, it is not "seemly" for seniors to cavort in the same fashion as do their children and grandchildren. Fortunately, we over sixty can make our own decisions on the matter. And do because it is a private affair. And that's just how I'm going to treat it here, as a private affair.

I have carried out interviews with a great many people in preparing this book, but I never felt like inquiring into their private sexual practices. Once in a while, someone volunteered a comment, but I didn't pursue the subject. The fact is that on television, in publishing, and in the newspapers we are awash in sexual information in the eighties. We're bombarded with the joy of sex. On the highways we see bumper stickers that proclaim "sailors make better lovers, joggers make better lovers, skiers make better lovers, coal miners make better lovers." How about "Eskimos make better lovers" or "Men with large hidden assets make better lovers"? I'm going to have some bumper stickers made up reading "Octagenarians make better lovers." I bet I'd sell a lot of those.

But seriously, I'm not going to cook up a long chapter on sex. If you want to know what percentage of seventy-year-olds have sex twice a week and which of the almost infinite varieties of copulation they prefer, there's sure to be a book someplace with that information. I just read in my daily paper that in a survey of twenty- to forty-year-olds, the average couple had sex six times a month. I don't know how reliable the survey was, but on converting it to weeks, I can't say I was deeply impressed by the youth of today. But I always have been impressed by that admirable courtesan of sixteenth-century France, Ninon de Lenclos, whose salon made an impact on the thinking of her times in both France and England and who is reputed to have had active lovers at least to the age of eighty. She then lived another ten years. Finally, in the middle of one night as she lay sleepless, she was moved to take a pad and pen she kept by her bedside and write the following words:

> Je suis en age de mourir
> Que ferois-je ici davantage?

My poor translation:

> I'm at the age of dying
> What better can I do here?

And at ninety she took leave of this world. Somehow this puts me in mind of another great French lady, a mover of history and a great lover of life, Eleanor of Aquitaine, who died four hundred years earlier in

Sex After Sixty

her eighty-third year. These French women of vitality seemed to know something about living long.

But what has all that got to do with sex? Probably very little. This is one area where I did go to the experts, rather than the practitioners And I got the same answer in every case. There are many who derive pleasure and an important dimension to their lives from engaging in sex into old age. There are just as many, probably more, who know intimacy, love, and relationships that lend a glow to their lives without sexual activity. That's what they say. And that's all I'm going to say.

12

Power

> Knowledge is power.
>
> —Bacon

Power—here is a word that over the centuries, has gathered evil connotations to itself. We think of the powers of evil. The powers that be. Lust for power. The corridors of power. The power of life and death. Power is always the ultimate ambition. But as is usually the case, there is another side to the coin. Give some thought to notions of power such as these.

> Power to heal.
> Power to teach.
> Power to enchant—through music, painting, other arts.
> Power to amuse.
> Power over oneself.
> Power to effect good.

The list could be extended to another page, but let me suggest just one more—Senior Power. A common picture of the elderly is one of people without power—powerless over where they live and how they live. They are seen as at the mercy of various social agencies, of their children, or of an unfeeling government at the state house or city hall.

There may be elements of truth in that dismal picture, but in the

LIFE BEGINS AT SIXTY

case of many senior citizens, the picture is quite different. The difference lies in how the affected individuals envision power. The one who sees himself as powerless almost certainly is so. The one who thinks he possesses power at least has a chance. The one who knows his power, understands where it lies, and also understands how to make use of it, that person actually has power over his own life and destiny.

I'm sure you'll remember Roy Hutchings, our former RAF ferry pilot, who is now an active wood sculptor. I wanted to talk to him about political power—Did he feel he had any? How had he used it, if ever? I know that senior citizens as a group possess a great deal of political power. You may have heard of the saying around Washington that "Social Security is like the third rail—touch it and you're dead!"

But what I wanted to explore here was political power at the individual and local level. In the small town in Connecticut where Hutchings has lived since coming to the United States, a recently formed committee, the Senior Citizen Tax Relief Committee, held a hearing at which Roy Hutchings, now an American citizen, spoke up. His question had to do with a property tax exemption of one thousand dollars for veterans, for which he had applied and been turned down. Admittedly he had not served in the U.S. forces, rather the RAF. But the way the town law now reads any *then* U.S. citizen who fought with an ally of the United States and also anyone who fought in the "free" Polish or Czechoslovakian forces (even though not a U.S. citizen) is eligible for the one thousand dollar exemption.

Does Roy Hutchings possess any political power? Two days after the Tax Relief Committee's meeting, he received a copy of a letter from the chairman to the appropriate town official requesting an amendment to the law that would make the tax exemption applicable to veterans of allied forces who were not then American citizens, but who now are. Action on the matter will take time, but there can be no doubt about the existence of Hutchings's political power expressed through the Senior Citizens Tax Relief Committee.

Does such a committee or instrument exist in your town or city? Is there any tax abatement program in effect for senior citizens? Do you

Power

think one is needed? What about neighboring localities? Can you find out how they stand on tax relief for the elderly? It will require just a few telephone calls for you to inform yourself on the situation.

Let's assume that you've made the calls and determined that your town is lagging in this matter. Answer me honestly. Do you feel like exercising your personal political power to change the situation and get tax relief for seniors where you live? Sounds like a big project, doesn't it? Maybe too much for one seventy-two-year-old lady or one seventy-eight-year-old man. It's not, if it's viewed as a series of little steps.

Try this scenario. You've decided that you, one person, are going to exercise your power to secure tax relief for seniors in your town. The first little step is just talk. Bring the subject up among your friends. Maybe you meet casually at a senior center or your church or on "Bingo" night. Tell your friends what you've found out about neighboring localities—how they are better off on taxes, and especially how they managed it. Pretty soon you'll have a nucleus of an interested group on tax abatement. No meetings, nothing formal, just a few persons who feel the tax situation, as it affects them, could be better.

At this point it's time to look for your "influential." This is a person whom you believe would make a good leader for your group and would represent you well in dealings with the appropriate local government officials. Again, you talk it up with your friends and reach agreement about trying to interest some individual in leading your effort. Is there a retired attorney among the seniors you know? Someone who held any position in government at the local level? Will he or she be interested in the aims of your group? Note that your power is not working alone now, but, rather, has extended itself to the six or eight friends who've been talking with you.

Now that you've all selected a potential leader and that person has agreed to at least look into the matter, things begin to get a little more formal. There'll probably be a meeting and discussion. And this is where you can choose your path—heavy involvement or little. You can simply let the group with its leader move ahead under its own momentum, restricting your role to that of "member of the group," and your power will continue to be effective both with the group or committee and the leader. Or you can jump on your horse and lead. In short you choose between being Don Quixote or Sancho Panza. In either case your own individual power will now begin to make itself felt.

Senior power working at the local government level is not only doable, but it's doable by you. Although he has been a tower of strength for seniors, Congressman Pepper, working for us in Washington, is not the only way in which senior political power works. For most of us the great barrier to exercising our political power, particularly at higher levels, is lack of knowledge. Honestly, can you name your representative in Washington? the names of the two senators from your state? Of course, voting is the first step in making yourself felt. Communication, usually by letter, is the next; and never underestimate that. Millions vote; thousands write—which means for a start that your letter is at least one thousand times as effective as a vote.

"Knowledge itself is power," Bacon's statement, at the head of this chapter reads. "Participatory citizenship knows no age barrier," Senator Lowell Weicker, Jr., of Connecticut said. Right. The only barrier is lack of knowledge, and toward overcoming that, Senator Weicker sponsors the Connecticut Senior Intern Program. Started eleven years ago, the program arranges for a five-day visit to Washington for senior citizens, organized around structured exposure to their government at work.

I asked Senator Weicker, who was a relatively young man when he started the program, what had moved him to do it. He replied, "Mother Bernadette of the Carmelite order, who is from Connecticut, saw my Junior Intern Program (which is for high school students) and said, 'Why don't you do something like it for senior citizens?' I sort of patted her on the head, patronized her, and said I thought it was a great idea and maybe we'd get around to it sometime. She just kept sitting on me, and all of a sudden we had it. So I give her credit for great persistence. She was on the Connecticut Council for Aging, and with her help we devised the program and it's been going ever since."

"Were your expectations fulfilled?" I asked.

"I think it's a great experience for the seniors. And you know it's been a great experience for my staff, too. When we started, we had some reservations. Number one, would the seniors get something useful out of it and enjoy themselves? Well, they have a blast! And number two has to do with my personal staff here in Washington. They're young, between twenty-five and thirty-five. And I think it's interesting to note that they look forward more to the senior program than to the junior program. There's a tremendous interaction between the seniors and the younger staff members. It's just terrific.

"They come down here," the senator continued, "and they learn and enjoy themselves. But, just as importantly, I think the younger people on my staff get a good perspective from a group of people who have a little experience and, frankly, do have something to say."

Incidentally, the program is not government funded; it is totally independent and paid for by substantial contributions from a very large number of corporations. As a result of the five-day visit to Washington, seniors find themselves equipped with the knowledge of how, and on whom, their political power should be used. As one put it, "Now we know where the buttons are and how to push them.

One senior who benefited from the five-day trip under the Senior Intern Program is Helen Imko, a registered nurse, sixty-eight years old, and a firm believer in using her own power wherever it can help the elderly. In the spring of 1982, the Reagan administration, through the Department of Health and Human Services, proposed an easing of nursing home regulations. On June 12, a news story in *The New York Times* by Robert Pear led off, "The Reagan administration's effort to change the rules for inspection of nursing homes is facing growing opposition." *The Times* continued, "Richard S. Schweiker, the secretary of health and human services, sought, for example, to drop the requirement for annual inspection of nursing homes." An articulate member of that "growing opposition" was our Helen Imko who immediately took the copybook action toward exerting her political power as a senior citizen. She wrote letters both to her senator, Lowell Weicker, Jr., and her representative, William R. Ratchford, member of Congress, fifth district, Connecticut. As a nurse

LIFE BEGINS AT SIXTY

who had on occasion worked in nursing homes, Imko did possess special knowledge, which she used along with newspaper clippings and other documentation in her letters to the two. Of course her visit to Washington under the Senior Intern Program was of great help because there she had met both the senator and the congressman personally.

That annual inspections of nursing homes was an important issue seemed obvious to Imko. There have been plenty of horror stories in the past about such facilities. Well, did she have any power? To answer that I'd like to quote from Senator Weicker's reply to her letter.

> Dear Mrs. Imko,
>
> Many thanks for your recent letter concerning care for the elderly—an issue which I too feel is of great national significance.
>
> [the next paragraph does not concern us, having to do with a book the senator tried to secure for Mrs. Imko.]
>
> I would also like to address the issue of nursing home deregulation. On May 27, 1982, the Department of Health and Human Services proposed the new regulations governing nursing homes that receive Medicare funding. I share the concerns many of my constituents have expressed regarding the proposed HHS regulations. Accordingly I have sent a letter to Secretary Schweiker, outlining my major objections to the new rules. A copy of this letter is enclosed.
>
> Again, I appreciate your contacting me on this matter and keeping me informed on your views.
>
> With kindest regards,
>
> Sincerely,
>
> Lowell Weicker, Jr.
> United States Senator

And what about Imko's congressman? I won't quote his full letter, which is lengthy, but these excerpts give an accurate picture of senior political power in action.

> Dear Ms. Imko,
>
> Thank you for your recent letter concerning a number of issues relating to the elderly. I also appreciate your sending me a number of articles and clippings, all of which were very informative.
>
> First I appreciate your support for my stand on the proposed easing of nursing home regulations.... I recently introduced House Concurrent Resolution 355, which expresses the sense of the Congress that regulations concerning the survey and certification of health care facilities participating in Federal Medicare and Medicaid programs should not be relaxed....
>
> [Here there were several paragraphs concerning other matters brought up by Mrs. Imko.]
>
> Once again I appreciate hearing from you. If I can be of any further assistance to you in any way, please do not hesitate to contact me again. I am thankful for your great support.
>
> Sincerely,
>
> William R. Ratchford
> Member of Congress
> Fifth District

Perhaps you will say, "Well, these are typical letters from politicians who just want to get reelected." But isn't that exactly the point? Of course, they want to get reelected; that's how our system works. The use of political power by any individual or group is based on, as Senator Weicker put it, "participatory citizenship." Incidentally, don't read these comments as suggesting that Weicker and Ratchford have as their only motivation the desire to get reelected. The records of both prove their sincere concern for the problems of the elderly. And the result of the political power exerted by Mrs. Imko and other seniors and other senators and congressmen is that the requirement for annual inspection of nursing homes was not dropped. Obviously, Imko's power was not the sole force behind defeating the effort at deregulation in this case. Everyone's power is limited, even the president's. Over the past two hundred years, every president has fumed at his inability to achieve certain objectives. The necessity of gathering the power of individuals toward achieving changes or improvements has always been a reality. Even President Reagan could not use his power effectively in the face of a hostile Congress.

Knowledge about political power is transferrable from the national to the state and local level. One of the objectives of the Connecticut Senior Intern Program is to educate seniors in such a way that they can take what they learn in Washington and go home and use it not only in the state capitol but in the operations of town government.

One senior who has done this effectively is Jane Forgacs, seventy years old, who lives in a little town in Connecticut. Following her five-day educational visit to Washington and meetings with her senators and congressmen, she came home and did exactly what the program had been designed for. First, she spread the word among those who had not made the trip. She wrote an interesting and informative lead article for the local weekly senior citizen's newspaper. Beyond that she spoke individually to as many seniors as possible. "I did my best to impress on them that they count. I told them from my own recent knowledge that what they think and say is heard in Washington. But I also told them that they will never be heard if they don't speak out. You know," she told me, "I've seen too many of our age group who feel isolated. And I had to tell them that we are growing in numbers and that we must get involved.

"And I was amazed," she continued vehemently, "at how many just felt the government didn't listen, that it was some impersonal object that simply acted as it wished."

"That's kind of unexpected," I said, "considering how much there seems to be in the news these days about the influence of older people on things like Social Security."

Power

"You'd be surprised," she replied, "at how isolated many old people are in their lives. So many of them narrow their circle of contacts down to their immediate families." I must admit that I had noticed something like that same phenomenon. Sure, people were aware of the great international tragedies, the hijackings, and so on; yet they were unaware of expenditures of millions of dollars, some of it their own money, within their own towns.

"Well, we stopped the Life Center the town tried to spend millions on against the will of the majority of seniors, didn't we?" Mrs. Forgacs referred to a planned conversion of an unused school into little apartments for the ambulatory elderly. The town government had been going ahead with little consultation with those most closely involved. When *they* studied the plans, they found many drawbacks to the planned conversion. Land had to be bought—expensive private property. The proximity to a thruway could be a danger to the elderly. So what did Mrs. Forgacs, with her Washington experience, do?

"Letters have to be written. Calls have to be made. Support has to be built up among the seniors. I wrote one letter to the paper that was published," she said with some quiet pride. "And together with all the seniors, we organized a referendum vote on the Life Center. Now I have to admit that we didn't get the full percentage needed to defeat the project, but the surprisingly large number voting against the construction of the Life Center so shocked the town government that eventually it was dropped. Of course, we still need it but in some other location and with more thorough planning."

"POWER. BOY, I can't even begin to describe the importance of power over oneself." So, Sylvia Greenfield Weiner of Ocean City, New York says. "To start out, being a diabetic I have to do thirty minutes of exercises every morning as soon as I get up. I can tell you I've never missed a day during the past fifteen years."

Mrs. Weiner was a social worker in New York City for most of her working life, finally becoming director of senior centers there. When she retired, she was certainly not willing to let all that experience go to waste, and she began to exercise a very personal power indeed by running classes, seminars, and consultations for those who have reached retirement age. She felt her life had given her a real sensitivity to what people who are about to retire need to know, and, with the help of Cornell University, she prepared a manual on pre-retirement training. Then she had an opportunity to test her ideas by working with the employees of the Republic Aircraft Company. Union and management in that company have arranged for employees nearing retirement to have time off during the day to attend sessions run by Mrs. Weiner.

"When I do the pre-retirement sessions and these blue collar workers look at me, they don't believe I'm seventy-three. And I have diabetes, basal-cell skin cancer, and arthritis. That lets me prove to them that having all these things doesn't make you a 'sick person.' I'm taking groups of from twenty to as many as three hundred people, and I'm grateful I have the energy. Why I've done a couple of thousand sessions over the past fifteen years.

"But I don't make this my whole life. I go to Florida for a couple of months every year, and I do a lot of other things. Fortunately, I still have my husband, but also, I have a great many women friends, old and young. And I find it marvelous to exchange ideas in the field of aging. Talking with the young can be very enlightening."

Here is a woman who exerts her influence in many areas. "Aside from Cornell and Republic Aircraft," she continued, "I've worked with civil service people. There's a lot of early retirement there, you know. They get bored with the unchanging routine, and advancement can be slow. Then I've worked with Local 237 of the Teamsters Union in New York, and I'll be doing some work for the Department of Health and Human Resources in December. I work for Adelphi University doing developmental aspects of aging, and I do a course here and there for the New School of Social Research in New York. I've also trained ombudspeople who go into nursing homes and actually work with the staff in nursing homes. My only hope is that I give people a lift."

Mrs. Weiner's bubbling vitality and cheerful manner raised my spirits during our interview and reminded me of my purpose in

Power

researching this book. Then, she said, "But you know, I'm feeling my aging now. I really am at seventy-three. My sixtieth birthday was nothing, but being seventy was a real knocker. They say seventy-five is when your decline is almost assured. But," she said with fire in her voice, "I'm going to fight that statistic a little bit." Sylvia Weiner has asked me to send her a copy of this book, which I certainly will. And I hope she draws as much strength as I have from meeting all the people in these pages who have demonstrated the power "to fight that statistic a little."

THE AMOUNT OF power you possess varies from one area to another. The range of its effectiveness extends all the way from practically nil over the actions of a Russian leader to extremely high, for example, over your personal health. An eight-year study conducted by researchers at Boston's Brigham and Women's Hospital shows that the average person possesses a high degree of control over his own health. Dr. Lee Goldman, director of the eight-year research, states that reduced smoking saved 150,000 lives during the period. George Burns may wave his cigar at millions on television and Eubie Blake may have smoked right up to the end, but the facts are that 150,000 people are now alive because they took power over their own health. Don't get me wrong here; I'm not trying to stop anyone from smoking (except at the next table in a restaurant). Everyone's life consists of continual trade-offs and it's up to you as an individual to make those decisions. It's how you live your life that makes it worth living. You have more than sixty years of experience filed in your brain. You have watched how others lived and have drawn your own conclusions. By now you know pretty well what is important in your life. So make your decisions based on all the factors involved.

I recently had to make a little decision of that sort myself. After my regular annual physical examination, my doctor was giving me the little wrap-up discussion that follows such events. He pointed out that, in general, everything was fine. "Your EKG is better than I've ever seen it." (I had a triple coronary bypass fourteen years ago.) "I suggest no butter, and it wouldn't hurt to lose a little weight."

LIFE BEGINS AT SIXTY

"No butter," I protested. "But I like good food, and butter is part of that." He gave me that blank look that seems to say, "It's your life, Buster." I walked out of his office with something to think about. Later I mentioned what he had said to my wife.

"Well, it wouldn't make that much difference," she said. "I cook with vegetable oil and about all we have is tubs of margarine."

"Is that what that is?" I thought I had been eating butter for years—slapping a good dollop into the frying pan whenever I fried an egg, splurging on butter on the english muffins in the morning. It slowly dawned on me that we had moved away from butter years ago. I then made the firm resolve not to eat butter. The next time I talked to the doctor I told him "You know it turns out that we almost never eat butter at home. We've been on low cholesterol margarine for some time—except perhaps for eating at restaurants."

"Good," he said with a faint smile. "That shouldn't be enough to do any harm."

Looking further at the eight-year study directed by Dr. Goldman, I see he reports that lower cholesterol intake was responsible for the saving of another 190,000 lives. I just took a deep breath and felt absolutely nothing in my chest. That's what I like to feel. But I did have one other feeling—a feeling of pleasure in the use of my own power to control my own health. Power over oneself. In the end, that may be the greatest form of power.

Here's another kind of power that I can't resist calling hobby power, and that brings us back to Roy Hutchings. Because of his happy years in Africa, Roy and his wife, Joyce, are always alert to news from that continent. Recently in their local newspaper, they saw an announcement of a luncheon to be given by the United Nations Association of the United States; a gathering whose purpose was to raise money to send two representatives to Africa for the purpose of organizing aid. The Hutchings were deeply touched by terrible scenes of starvation in Africa and Roy's response was to donate a life-size wood sculpture of a short-billed dowitcher, a water bird normally seen on beaches and mud flats of the Eastern United States, for raffling at the U.N. Association meeting. The accurately and beautifully painted replica of this shore bird will probably bring eighty-five dollars to one hundred dollars at auction.

Later I wanted to translate Roy's hobby power into the realistics of its effect on people actually facing death in Africa. So I called the local chapter of "Save-the-Children International" to ascertain what the effective power of Roy's dowitcher (at one hundred dollars) would be. Listen to this. The power of one man's gift of twenty-five to thirty hours of work in his basement will feed ten children for two hundred days or close to seven months. The look on Roy's face and the tone his voice took on when I told him of the figures supplied by "Save-the-Children" was all the evidence I'll ever need to demonstrate the value to oneself of using an apparently minor power in the right way.

FROM "HOBBY" POWER to power over oneself, to political power—they're all efforts to exert control. The struggle for power of any and every kind seems almost to characterize the history of humankind. In fact, the drive to exert power over its environment seems to characterize life itself. From the one-celled paramecium moving something edible toward its "mouth" by means of its cilia, to the cancer cell growing wild at the expense of its neighbors, to the farmer plowing a field to do his will—even the months-old baby screaming defiance at a world that won't respond to his will—all life seems determined to bend the environment and its fellow creatures to its will. Yet as sure as God made little fishes, all of us, from the single-celled guys to the great dictators, eventually come up against a situation in which we cannot prevail. Like Sisyphus, no matter how many times we push the boulder to the top of the hill, it rolls back down again. And this brings us smack up against one of the most important aspects of power—the situation in which we find we are powerless. How one responds to that may be one of the secrets of enjoying life at any age.

Here's a lady, in her middle eighties, one of the most engaging, lively, enjoyable people I've talked with in researching this book. I'm going to call her "Ruth"; that's not her name but that's what she asked me to do. Ruth has probably had a little more than her share of power during a long, active, and effective life. Perhaps for exactly that reason, I chose her for this question. "Have you ever faced a situation, of importance, you could not control—where you were powerless—and how did you handle that?"

"I've surely had some baffling things to meet," she replied, "but usually life went on—I found some way to handle them. But, well..." she hesitated, "I guess the most traumatic thing I ever had to do was ... well, I was already into my sixties, and it turned out that my husband of many years became an alcoholic. I'll tell you this. Read the books, see the movies, maybe you'll get a faint idea. But the real thing—it has to be lived. Talk about not having power." Ruth paused a minute, something of a frown on her face. "He was an actor, not a leading man, but a fine character actor." She smiled. "Remember what they call the golden age of television? The fifties and the sixties? Well, if you watched *Studio One* or *Armstrong's Circle Theater* and others like that, you've probably seen him. He came back after the war—he was a pilot flying in Europe, Distinguished Flying Cross and all that—and then, he succeeded in acting almost right away. We bought a house in Connecticut. I was an ad executive with one of the big agencies, and life was looking pretty good. And we both liked our drinks—it was part of that life. I think I enjoyed them as much as he did. But then, after awhile, I began to think there was something different. For example, he'd have to have a couple before we went out to a party and a lot after we got home at night, too."

"Did you try to do something about it?" I asked.

"That was the stone wall," she said. "That's where you just can't tell a man anything—or a woman, I suppose. I certainly didn't have any control there."

"But you kept trying?"

"Well, that was just it. Everything would be fine for a while, so it looked as though I was wrong. But finally, it was really obvious. He stopped acting completely. I'd commute into New York and worry all day about what would happen before I got back."

"What—did he get so he couldn't go in front of the cameras?"

"No. They'd call him up for jobs, and he'd turn them down. He just didn't go in."

"Did you try to get him to go to AA or to see anyone?" I asked.

"He would do nothing about it. I went to psychiatrists and consultants, and they tried to help me know how to get him to go. I knew that unless he did something, nothing would happen."

"I'm not trying to lead you, Ruth, but would you say you were powerless at that point?"

"No, I kept trying. I went to our regular doctor, and he knew I wanted to have help. He sent me to a psychiatrist who would be able to help me. But 'I'm not sick' that's all my husband would say, and he wouldn't do any of the things that were suggested by the doctor. I guess all the power I had wasn't enough. It came to where I finally had to divorce him. It had to be two lives or none."

"I don't understand."

"I didn't have any life. I knew I'd never have a life if I stayed with him. I still loved the guy I married—but the guy I married wasn't there. So I took our bank account, everything, and I divided it and gave him half—in the lawyer's office, of course. And I said, 'Now you're on your own.' Seeing that man sitting there in the lawyer's office, crying—that was probably the most traumatic thing I ever had to do."

I waited a minute in the silence and then asked, "How did you feel when you took that step?"

"Relief, I guess, later. It took awhile. I don't think I thought of it as relief for some time. Then when it struck me, finally, it was like a flood. I was washed in relief. The weight was lifted off me. I don't think I ever experienced such a feeling of freedom. It was just not my responsibility anymore. Really, I had wings. This happened in October, and it wasn't until December that I could get my affairs and job responsibilities straight enough to take a trip to the Orient in order to really get my mind straightened out . . . a completely different atmosphere."

I asked, "Was the trip a good idea?"

"Oh yes, I've been healthy ever since. I'm a bitch, you know. I won't let anything cheat me out of a good life. Also, I had my work, I had lots of friends, and I had the house. I just picked up a new life."

LIFE BEGINS AT SIXTY

Now, in her eighties, Ruth still has a good life. It's full of friends, full of activities—intellectual and physical—and she finds time and energy to do some important good things for other people as well. As for the actor, he went through the money, a stay in a veteran's hospital, and his life, all in short order.

Where did the power lie in all of this? Ruth found that she didn't have it. There was no way she could control the situation. The husband? Well, he wouldn't admit his powerlessness. But Ruth did what we all have to do when we finally are forced to conclude that we don't have power to control a situation. She let go. She turned it over to God or the force or destiny—however you want to characterize it.

WE'VE BEEN TALKING about different kinds of power possessed by older people. One of the finest kinds of power is the power to make people feel good—to make people happy. Be sure to work that one into your schedule. But take note also of the fact that using power makes the user feel good. There's a glorious feeling about stepping down hard on the accelerator, feeling the surge of power as the car accelerates. Then there's the power to make people laugh. It is perhaps one of the most satisfying—to see your listeners doubled up, faces distorted in hilarity, yet distorted into a happy caricature. That affords the storyteller an almost divine pleasure. Watch the face of Buddy Hackett as he watches his audience just after he has gotten off a particularly good one.

There are so many kinds of power and, probably, as many ways of using it for good or to give pleasure as there are for evil. Money is another obvious source of power, and it, as much as anything, can surely be used for good or ill. I remember my mother once saying, with a smile, "There's one thing about having money, it keeps you close to your children."

Why don't you make an inventory of the various kinds of power you possess? Don't make it a big job or write a list; just noodle the concept. As the various powers come to mind, think specifically about when you last made use of that particular one. Could you have used it more

Power

often? Would it, perhaps, be useful to you today? Specifically, how did it make you feel—using that power? Remember

> Senior Power is good power;
> Senior Power has many faces;
> Senior Power is good for seniors.

13

Keep Moving

We do not count a man's years until he has nothing else to count.
—Emerson

One day, during my freshman year at college, the same biology professor who kept the long-lived amoeba in his watch fob, was trying to develop some simple definition of life that we sixteen- and seventeen-year-olds could comprehend. "Look for movement," he said. "Movement generally signifies life just as a complete lack of movement characterizes death." So my sincere advice to anybody over sixty is to "keep moving," and that's how I picked the title for this chapter.

I CAN HARDLY think of anyone who typified that advice better than Dora Spangler of Wichita, Kansas. After bringing up four children and guiding many grandchildren, Mrs. Spangler decided she needed more activity in her life. So back in the 1960s and at the age of 82, she took up golf. She was also an avid bowler, but eventually she decided the sport was too much for her, and she retired from the lanes at 100. She continued as a familiar figure on the local golf courses until, at 103, she concluded that at 79 pounds she was a little fragile for golf. "I guess I'll have to take up crocheting," she said. After two years of plying the needles, this admirable lady died just over a year ago at 105.

After that, a 74-year-old commercial pilot may sound a bit youthful.

LIFE BEGINS AT SIXTY

And if the way he wracks his open biplane around is any yardstick, you might well call Bob Gunn a young pilot.

"I STARTED FLYIN'" in 1928, the day after Hoover was elected, and I've been flyin' ever since." Bob Gunn has without a doubt kept moving all of his seventy-three years. Fifty-seven years ago, he was learning to fly in an old Eagle Rock biplane. Forty-four years ago, he was flying Lockheed Hudson bombers across the North Atlantic for the beleaguered Royal Air Force; and this year, he is flying single-engine Piper Pawnees, crop dusting something like a thousand acres a day. Bob lives with his wife in Tchula, Mississippi, and has been flying for a living since the mid-1930s, alternating teaching flying with crop dusting. "I've got two children, six grandchildren—two of 'em's already graduated from college," he told me with quiet pride in his voice, "and one is a lieutenant in the air force out at Vandenberg Air Force Base on the coast."

If I ever heard what it is that made America great, it was what he was telling me. He ferried uncounted twin- and four-engine bombers for RAF Ferry Command in the effort to destroy Hitler; once he lost an engine over the Mediterranean taking a Halifax from England to Cairo; he taught the art of flying to several hundred young men, perhaps with dreams like his own; he made his quiet contribution to the agriculture of the South for about fifty years (and still does) while at the same time caring for a family. He won't be president of the United States, but without citizens like Bob Gunn, a president wouldn't have much to work with.

And if work isn't enough to keep Gunn moving, he's chief cook and bottle washer on the home front, too. "My wife's got arthritis real bad," he told me. "She's in a wheelchair most of the time. So I do all the cookin' and house cleaning and washing and everything. That's the reason I don't have much time for recreation." Money didn't seem to be a problem for Gunn, so I asked him why he was still flying—a job that consumed many hours and held not a little danger.

"I gotta have something to do," he said in what seemed a nonsequitur. "I can't just set around." Flying, I began to think, might just be

Keep Moving

Gunn's recreation. He laughed at my question. "I just like the way they fly—gettin' up there where nobody bothers you."

I've seen a few pictures of crop-dusting airplanes, as I guess we all have, whipping along four or five feet above the plants they're spraying, pulling up just enough to miss the utility wires at the ends of the fields, and I've often wondered about those wires. If you saw the newsreel pictures of Lindbergh's take-off for his nonstop flight to Paris in 1927, you'll remember one of the most striking things was the way his overloaded *Spirit of St. Louis* barely cleared the wires at the end of Floyd Bennett Field. Ten feet lower and the flight probably would have ended in a ball of fire right there. I asked Gunn about the threat posed by the wires. "We got wire cutters on these Pawnees," he said. "They got wire cutters on the landing gear, and then there's one right up in front of the windshield, and of course, your propeller's going to do a pretty good job of cutting, too."

"Have you ever hit the wires?" I asked.

"Oh, I've been through some wires and stuff," he laughed, "but it didn't bother me. I've done a little damage, but I've never had to go down."

"But what about the electricity from the wires? Some of them carry pretty high voltage?"

He laughed heartily at that. "Oh, yeah. Plenty of sparks, a lot of flashing, but those planes go through anything. The only thing about running through the wire is if it wraps around something—that brings you down. If it cuts clean, why you don't have too much trouble."

There's a very old saying in the world of flying, and it goes like this: "There are old pilots, and there are bold pilots; but there are no old, bold pilots." I began to wonder—maybe I had found one. I asked him how many flying hours he had.

"I've got a little over 24,000 hours," he said.

Then I asked about how his health had been over the past seventy-three years. "Health?" he said as if I had mentioned something that took place on Saturn. "Fine. I never had any trouble. I had a little bit of arthritis about four years ago. I had a little pain in my shoulder, and

LIFE BEGINS AT SIXTY

I thought I'd just pulled it. Went to my wife's arthritis doctor, and they found a vertebrae in my neck that was causing the pain. So he gave me some exercises to take, and after about a month, it went away. And I take the exercises every day, and I haven't had any more trouble. Don't take any medicine at all."

"What about age and your pilot's license?" I asked.

"Age doesn't matter," he said. "As long as you can pass the physical. I've got a commercial license."

"What was it like, learning back in the twenties?"

"Oh, there was a fella come around every week. Then sometimes he couldn't get around for two or three weeks. Then he'd give you an hour or seventy minutes. Didn't take long. It wasn't that complicated back then, you know."

I was still thinking about 24,000 hours! I can't quite comprehend that much time in the air. And Gunn wasn't sitting there behind an automatic pilot monitoring a panel of instruments the way flying is for so many pilots today. That's 24,000 hours of full attention, much of it at an altitude of ten to twenty feet! That's, of course, excepting the crossing of the North Atlantic at any altitude and in any weather, night and day during wartime.

As I concluded my interview with Gunn, he told me he was leaving Mississippi in a few days to spend a couple of months with his sister and family in Black Canyon, Arizona. "We just park our motor home in their backyard," he said. "Motor home"—I should have known. This man's middle name should be "mobile."

Was there anything he'd like to say to his fellow seniors reading this book? He laughed his usual chuckle. "One of my little granddaughters—she's in first year high school—she says, 'Get with it.'"

HOW MUCH FURTHER from the skies over the cottonfields of Mississippi can you go than to the interiors of a museum? That's a measure of the difference between the lives of Bob Gunn and Walter Long. Yet both of these men are prime examples of people who have "kept moving." Born in 1904, Walter K. Long has been director of the Cayuga Museum of History and Art in Auburn, New York, since 1936, when

Keep Moving

he secured the building and founded the museum. Now eighty-one, Long runs the museum with one secretary and a couple of young assistants, although he mounts as many as seven and more major shows each year. In addition he travels widely, securing materials for the exhibitions and fulfilling his obligations as member of the International Council of Museums of UNESCO, and teaching and lecturing at universities here and abroad. Professor Long is, by my own observations, a veritable whirlwind of activity. If there can be a perfect example of the meaning of this chapter, "Keep Moving," Long is it.

When I asked him the other day about his level of activity in his eighty-second year, he said, "Well, I don't get up until around seven-thirty, but I'm at work at the museum by nine and should be through by five, unless there's an event in the evening—camera club meeting or such like. But, I'll tell you, I've just lost two people and these days I'm going until eleven o'clock as often as not." Generally, there are what Long calls "events" four evenings a week, such as the camera club or the "Daubers" as the art group is known. The Cayuga Museum was built as a Greek revival mansion in 1836. Now, as a museum, it has four large display rooms and a gift shop on the main floor, smaller display rooms and offices on the second floor, and permanent storage on the third floor and in the basement. In addition there are two outbuildings, a long converted greenhouse that is now an art studio for painting and sculpture, and a large old-fashioned barn in which a stage for dance and a second floor for housing permanent collections have been built. Long supervises everything with the help of volunteers.

I can't tell you all of Long's activities since graduating from Syracuse University in the twenties, but he is an expert in such diverse fields as painting, sculpture, architecture, history, archeology, and drama. Perhaps his best known work was in translating the small models sculpted by Gutzon Borglum for the Mount Rushmore National Monument into the actual sixty-foot busts we see today. I'll tell you more about the twelve-year task later. At age sixty-nine he had a heart attack and underwent bypass surgery but managed to get back on the job at the museum within a couple of months.

LIFE BEGINS AT SIXTY

I asked this energetic octogenarian what plans he had for the museum in the current year. "Oh, this is going to be a big year," he said characteristically. "For instance, the first show, just coming up, is 'What Is Abstract?' And I'll try to make it clear to people the different 'isms' that led to our postabstract painting. That's March."

I asked how many different exhibitions there would be in the year.

"There'll be three major exhibitions this spring. Then, we have our usual big show, which lasts two months in the summer. Then for the fall I have three other major exhibitions scheduled. Now, after the abstract show, we have a one-man show coming of a local artist who's gaining national recognition. That'll be followed by a big photography show. Along with the big shows, there'll be smaller shows: painting shows, drawing shows, print shows, and smaller photography shows."

I couldn't stop the flow of coming attractions. "After the big summer show, the first fall show is 'Wells Fargo and the Great Western Movement.' We'll play up the pony express as an exhibit and feature all western paintings, showing the western art of the time and early western days. The second fall show is 'Folk Art' showing the period of 1800 to 1825. It will illustrate what happened in that period, how they worked, what their tools were, and so on. Oh, I forgot, in late November comes the 'Dollerama,' one of the most interesting collections of historical American dolls—and that's one that brings the children in. You know it's important to get them young and build their interest in what's to be found in a museum."

"How about travel?" I asked.

"Oh yes, I take many trips. Now, for instance, in the next ten days I'll be making three trips for the next exhibition. One of them is to Hyde Park to pick up some Waughs [Frederick Waugh]. Yes, for every exhibition I make trips to bring the show in and handle it. No, I don't hang pictures myself," he answered my raised eyebrows, "I have one boy who's an intern. He's healthy and strong, does the lifting and hanging after I've determined where they're going."

"Do you have time for vacations?" I asked.

"Well, last year we went to Hawaii. We couldn't get all the children together, so we went to Hawaii and had our first Christmas alone." Long has a wife, three children and many grandchildren, and even one great-granddaughter.

"Any vacation since?" I asked.

"No," he laughed. "I'm not planning anything until I get this business on the road. So probably in the spring, I'll start thinking."

I marveled at his ability to juggle so many projects at the same time, as well as handling visitors to the museum. "I depend on a large volunteer group—we call them 'docents'—who take people around, handle traffic, and so forth." I later had to go to my dictionary for "docents"; it was there all right. "Lecturers, guides," Webster said. "Now, tomorrow night," Long hurried on, "I'm starting a new group. I've got a good instructor here, and the young will be learning to do small pieces of carving. You know, I want to attract those youths who whittle—maybe with a jackknife."

I want to interrupt the professor's flow of words a moment to tell you something about his health. Unlike our crop duster Bob Gunn, Long has not lived a life of perfect health. His major problem came at the age of sixty-nine. In Long's own words: "I had a little heart disturbance twelve years ago, but it wasn't a serious heart attack. Part of a vessel had blown up like a balloon, but luckily, it didn't burst. They managed to get me to the hospital soon enough, and I had an operation. They put in a dacron tube to replace the damaged artery."

"How long were you out of action?" I asked.

"I don't know—two, maybe three months. But as soon as I could, I made a sort of office out of the hospital room. Everybody came in there, and we did business. There were a few weeks like that."

"So, it didn't affect your career?"

"Oh, no, not at all," Long said firmly. "If anything, it made me anxious to do more, and I have been doing more."

"How are you feeling these days?" I asked.

"Terrific! I say that because I've had two or three little things that are very bothersome, but I know they're things that will soon be over and I can forget them. For example, my foot—it was cut badly. Now, the bandages will be coming off completely in two or three days. You see, I was working with the display cases here. I was down behind one, and I got up in a hurry. The case ripped across my foot, and I pulled the tendons at the same time." Long spent several days in bed, but you can be sure he was back at work as soon as the doctor let him go.

I mention Long's health because it's so important to recognize that it's not what *happens to us* that's so important as *how we handle* the event. "Keep moving" seems to have been Long's motto ever since he came out of college. It was shortly after graduating that he came in contact with Gutzon Borglum because of an interest in sculpture. They worked together on the figures at Stone Mountain in Georgia; and then, off and on from 1929 to 1941, Long was deeply involved in the work at Mount Rushmore, where the four massive presidential busts now gaze across the Black Hills.

"If you look up my name on the project you'll see I'm described as 'Pointer.' You see I had to figure out from the small busts in the studio where, on the mountain face, each characteristic of the face would be located—the chin, eyes, nose, and so forth. First, it was a matter of rough sculpting with dynamite, before getting down to the fine work that was done with drills and the like."

"How did you get that job?" I asked. "You were pretty young then, weren't you?"

"Borglum had seen some of my sculpture," he replied, "and he recognized the fact that I was always looking for projections that would catch light and create shadows. So what we did to get them up on the mountain was to mount a large boom on top of each head so that it could swing back and forth over a big protractor, showing degrees. At ninety degrees the boom would be right over the nose, the center of the bust and the chin. I had a similar setup on the sixty-inch models in the studio, and any point on the final sculpture could be found by three numbers—the number of degrees to which the boom swung, the number of feet out horizontally on the boom, and the number of vertical feet down from that spot on the boom. That's how I transferred the tip of the nose on the sixty-inch model to the tip of the nose on the mountain itself. Only on the mountain it was feet instead of inches.

Keep Moving

"But you can imagine there were hundreds of 'points' that had to be calculated for the four presidential heads. I made them up in what I called 'point books.' For every inch on the sixty-inch model, I created four 'points' that, when enlarged to feet on the mountain, actually shaped the faces. So they worked from my book to get to each point—which is why I was called 'Pointer.'"

"Did you ever work on the mountain?" I asked.

"No. That was dynamiting and drilling. The workers used dynamite to get down to within a few feet of the 'point,' then they used drills and finer tools. But you know when you get up on the mountain and you stand on the nose, you can't see anything. You stand there on the nose, and you can't see the sides of the face at all. You can't see the chin at all. You can't see the forehead."

"Did you really get out and stand on the nose?"

"Oh, many times."

"Did you have safety harnesses?"

"Yes. They were like—you strapped yourself into a seat and a five-eighths-inch steel cable ran down from the top. Of course, I was in my thirties then. But I didn't spend much time there once my 'point books' were done. Although I did go back often to see how it was coming. Then, of course, I started the museum in 1936. But, do you know how it all ended? It was almost done in 1941. But that year, when Mr. Borglum died, you see, we all got together and we said, 'This is it. The monument stops right here.' So we left it—took all the cables and the protractors, took down the houses on top of the heads, and the booms, and so on. The idea was this is just the way Mr. Borglum left it."

For a moment I was reminded of Dr. Gilbert Leib when the time came for the amputation of his leg. "You've got to know when to say 'Good-bye,'" he had said. And here Long and the others had known the right time to say good-bye to Mount Rushmore, leaving it just where Gutzon Borglum left it.

Walter Long has faced plenty of setbacks in his eighty-odd years though. One took place in his seventieth year, when the museum was set on fire by careless painters using blowtorches. Water from fire hoses nearly ruined the entire collection of books and paintings. But with his usual élan, Long inspired more than three hundred emergency volunteers to pitch in, place absorbent paper between the pages of all the books; and then, he quick froze them all in volunteered freezers. This halted mildew until he could build a "thymol" oven that could get rid of what mildew had occurred. Paintings are taking longer because of the expertise needed in restoration, but the museum was back in business in a matter of months. I was not too surprised to learn that all the local restaurants in the small town had provided free food and drink for the volunteers during the emergency period. Quick action and unbridled enthusiasm just seem to attract the same in others near the situation.

"So what lies ahead now?" I asked Long as the interview wound down.

"Now after this year we're in now when I'm emphasizing history, art activity, and conservation—this year with the intense program, is actually preparing for the really big year—the museum's fiftieth birthday next year. Then I'm planning a different kind of exhibit, a more or less permanent exhibit. But in the fall I'll get together examples of all the artists I've borrowed from over the years, and that's going to celebrate our fiftieth birthday—fifty years since I started the place as director.

"You know," he said in an afterthought, "when I started this museum, I purposely made it flexible. In other words, I didn't have to sit here every day. And I went out and I did sculpture and paintings and portraits, and I did mosaics and frescoes and things like that."

As a parting shot, Long mentioned, "Strangely enough I got a commission to do a little portrait today." The portrait turned out to be of Harriet Tubman, the escaped slave, who in pre-Civil War days organized the "underground railway" that runaway slaves used to make their way from one "safe house" to another and north to freedom. "She came here after she got through with her work in New Jersey," he continued, "but all her pictures were taken when she was in her eighties and nineties, shortly before she died in 1913—she looks old and ugly. I didn't like the idea of painting her like that—after all, she was young when she did her work. So I decided to paint her when she was young, vibrant, and really working for the black race."

"How are you going to do that?" I asked.

"I will do it by taking the characteristic parts of her face and retrogressing to what they would have been. I'm planning to get her when she was about thirty-two." I have seen the usual pictures of Harriet Tubman, and I don't mind saying I'm really curious to see what Long's portrait will look like. It occurs to me that what he is doing is not entirely unlike the transformation of the sixty-inch models of the presidents to the sixty-foot busts on Mount Rushmore.

YOU KNOW "KEEP moving" can refer to something purely physical, as it does in the case of Steve Bekasi, now seventy-seven years old, who puts in a full season of ice hockey and has been doing so for probably more than fifty years. "Hawk," as he is known to his younger competitors, earned his nickname by the way he swooped from nowhere to steal the puck.

I asked him about the age of the others with whom he competed in one of the roughest games around. "Oh, some of them are in their teens, some in their twenties—there are even some up in their forties!"

"Why do you take that kind of punishment?" I asked.

"That's no punishment. I do it because the activity makes me feel good. It makes me feel good physically and mentally—just as simple as that."

LET'S GO BACK into the wild blue yonder once more with one of American aviation's most active female flyers, Nancy Hopkins Tier. Like Bob Gunn, she soloed in 1927, but she celebrated Hoover's election by flying low over the inaugural parade up Pennsylvania Avenue—an action, she said, "that probably had something to do with the passage of laws against low flying in built-up areas." Tier is one of three members still flying of the original "Ninety-Nines," an association formed in 1929 of ninety-nine female pilots, which included such illustrious names as Anne Morrow Lindbergh and Amelia Earhart.

LIFE BEGINS AT SIXTY

Does she, now at the age of seventy-six, still keep moving? Failing to reach her for several days, I finally found her at home on a Tuesday afternoon. She had flown home the previous Sunday evening from a meeting in Baltimore on aviation business. "Monday morning," she explained, "I flew up to Vermont to get my dog—my eldest son had been keeping him for me—then back to Lakeville the same night to meet two friends. We're planning a monthlong tour of Wales for next month. Then, in a couple of days, I'll be flying to Lake George, New York, where we spend our summers." When I said I felt lucky to have caught her, she replied, "Well, you just caught me. When the phone rang, I had just come in from cutting the lawn, and now, I've got to run to the post office to get this letter off to Wales about our trip." Whereupon this thoughtful lady gave me a one-hour interview on the spot.

We talked about the early days of flying for a bit, and then I brought up the matter of age. "I don't relate to my age in any way to tell you the truth. I know the number is seventy-six, but it doesn't seem to have anything to do with me—if you can see what I mean?" I did. "Every once in awhile, I think about it. Well, to have the perspective on life that you get when you get older, that's a wonderful kind of interesting thing, as well as still being able to take advantage of all the fun that's available today."

One part of her life that gives Nancy Tier perspective on both life and flying is the period during World War II when she flew as a member of the Civil Air Patrol (CAP), spotting German U-boats off the U.S. East Coast. When we first entered the war, the Germans practically had carte blanche right up to our shores, sinking as many as three or four ships per night. But after the Civil Air Patrol flooded the area, the many civilian pilots swelling the numbers of Navy and Coast Guard patrols, sinkings eventually dropped by as much as eighty percent.

Having joined the Civil Air Patrol in 1942 and served by flying off the coast of Maine through the war, Mrs. Tier became the first female wing commander in Connecticut—a post she held for four years until she was named colonel in the CAP. She is still very active in the Civil

Keep Moving

Air Patrol, but her major project is directing and aiding the construction of the International Women's Air and Space Museum, now coming into existence in Dayton, Ohio. The complex will commemorate women like Anne Lindbergh, Nancy Love, and Amelia Earhart, who made substantial contributions to the growth of aviation.

"What are you flying now?" I asked, curious as to the choice of such an experienced flyer.

"A Cessna 170 'tail dragger,'" she replied, referring to the single tail wheel, which may seem a little old-fashioned today. "It fills my needs now, and I can afford to fly it. You know it saddens me to see so many pilots buy some of the wonderful new airplanes and then find that the cost of gas and maintenance cripples what they can do."

But Mrs. Tier is not always in the air. One of her favorite activities is serving as a volunteer in nursing homes near where she lives. She says patients particularly respond when she reads to them from books about and by women aviators. "There's something about flying that appeals to the spirit and spirituality of most of us," says Mrs. Tier, who is also a bible school teacher and active member of her church.

Flying has always been special to me and so I'm always interested in what it means to other pilots. I asked the inevitable question: "What is it that you like about flying, Mrs. Tier?"

"I feel very strongly that man has probably wanted to fly ever since he watched the first bird take off. And in all of time, it's only been in this century—my lifetime, really—that man has been able to fly. I think it's one of the great privileges of living—an incredible thing to be able to do—and to do it yourself. I particularly love to be able to fly myself around and observe the earth from low altitudes.

"The beauty of the sky just passes anything. And clouds—my friends think I'm a nut for all the pictures I take of clouds. Seeing them from above, of course, is something you can never see from the earth. And under certain conditions—a storm breaking out, lightning from above. And another thing, the whole earth looks so peaceful from a few thousand feet. It looks so good, beautiful, and at peace. You just have to wonder why people are scrapping and cutting each other's throats down there."

LIFE BEGINS AT SIXTY

Mrs. Tier clearly has an attitude toward both life and death that grows out of a deep spirituality. Referring to the early days, she says, "We flew with virtually no equipment, no brakes, no radio, three very simple instruments, and a very uncertain engine. I had six forced landings before I was thirty, and I believe strongly in Divine Providence—that I'm still around because he has some purpose for me. The big world is the world of the spirit," she stated, "and I do believe it's going to be exciting, the next step."

AS YOU READ these pages, I'm going to ask you to reminisce with me a little over all the people you've been reading about. They are just a few of the millions who have entered "the Living years" and who are making the best out of each day of their lives. Think of Barbara Coburn preparing to enter the water of Southport Harbor. Or think of eighty-eight-year-old Ernie Systrom stepping out on the golf course again, holding a club with his self-rejuvenated hands. I could go on, but you know the people I'm talking about. And what they offer is proof that sixty is nothing but an imaginary line with about as much significance as the line between two time zones. Life offers the same challenges and the same satisfactions on either side. I must echo Bob Gunn's "little granddaughter," who says, "Get with it." She's talking to you and me.

But if you happen to be one of those who's not totally "with it," getting there means change, an activity most of us have resisted since birth. "Objects at rest tend to remain at rest," Sir Isaac Newton said. Yet, as we've seen, exceptions are many. And the other half of Newton's law says, "Objects in motion tend to remain in motion. Once you get "in motion," you'll tend to continue that way.

Getting in motion. No more difficult step will face you than that one. If some of the people in this book have interested you, why then go back to the chapter they're in and look at their story. Once you've found one who moves you to think: "Gee, maybe I could . . . ," then, take the advice of one Mississippi teenager and "get with it."

14

Enjoy

Of a good beginning cometh a good end.
—John Heywood

As we approach the end of what, for me, has been a pleasant, sometimes exciting, and always enlightening journey through the lives of a group of people especially blessed with the ability to savor life as most do not, I hope you will turn a gently critical eye on your own life. Don't be put off by the word "critical." The purpose of a critique is to improve something. "How's the soup? Mmm, I think it could do with a little more salt." Maybe your life—maybe my life—could do with a little more salt. There they all are, in these pages, real-live everyday people, just like you and me in most respects. But these people, for the reasons we've seen, like the existence of variety in their days, having clear-cut goals that power their lives, knowing and utilizing the power they possess, tasting the satisfactions of doing good things for others, and all the other qualities of life we've explored; these people *are* different. For one thing, they are living longer than their brothers and sisters. For another, the quality of their days is so superior that I estimate it ranks up there with the top 10 percent of the population at any age. That proves to me that we over-sixties have no reason in the world to settle for a life in any degree less happy, or less satisfying, than the under-sixties.

Quality of time. A concept I've never given much thought to before.

LIFE BEGINS AT SIXTY

Air quality—we talk about that all the time. There are days in Los Angeles when the word quality should not appear in the same sentence as air. Crossing the North Atlantic by ship, I can remember days when the quality of the air was truly "like wine," when to inhale a deep lungful of that ocean-washed substance truly made one feel giddy, truly sent the spirit soaring. The quality of time too can be like wine. Right now it's possible that Bob Gunn may be taxiing out to take off for a day's crop dusting. As an old pilot, I will dare to say that I know something of how he feels. Hand on the throttle of his Piper Pawnee, he uses a light touch on the foot brake to swing straight on the runway, and then, he quickly but smoothly pushes the throttle wide open and locks it. Acceleration is rapid and he sinks back into the seat as the plane rapidly gathers speed. There is a slight crosswind and the aircraft fights it as the pilot uses rudder to hold straight down the runway. The hard ground transmits its roughness to the pilot's body, particularly when the wheels bounce a little sideways in that crosswind. Then, at a certain moment, the craft becomes airborne— borne by air alone as it gently sways, sinks, and rises in the early morning currents. The ground drops away and is quickly forgotten. Green cottonfields of Mississippi become three-dimensional as the craft gains altitude and the horizon becomes a straight line as mariners always see it. Throttling back to "cruise" he takes up a course toward the day's work. If Bob Gunn is like me, he probably starts singing at this point. As Gunn put it, "Well, you're up there alone— where nobody can bother you." Yet one is not up there alone; one is never really alone. It's just that the grime, the noise, and all the warts of earthbound life are missing. One has a look at the earth as it was created. I would say that the quality of Bob Gunn's time, at age seventy-four, in the air over Mississippi, is of a very high order indeed.

Or let's take that morning when Ruby Hemenway sat in the sunny window of her little house in Turners Falls, at the age of ninety-nine, and started writing the following words for next week's "I Remember When" column:

Enjoy

Sometimes, in a large formal garden, you will find a sun dial. These days they are purely ornamental and do not have the practical use they once had. But sometimes early settlers found just where the sun was at noon and made a mark on their door sill. That mark was called the "noon mark" and it was all the time piece they had.

One of the earliest clocks a householder could afford was a very simple one that hung on the wall of the large kitchen that served as living quarters for the entire family. It was called a "Wag on the Wall" with the simplest works possible, a face painted with the figures—not Roman numerals—and often with two crudely done pictures in the upper corners. The works at first were not even enclosed in a case, and there was a long pendulum with a flat metal disc on the end and a cat gut cord holding a heavy sealed cylinder of sand.

When the clock was wound (Sunday morning) that weight was pulled up, then let down tick by tick during the week so it made a pleasant, companionable, unhurried sound—"tick, tock, tick, tock."*

While writing her column on time-keeping in New England in the early days, Hemenway undoubtedly enjoyed the events brought to mind by the family "wag on the wall," the image of her father winding it Sunday mornings and who knows what other pictures from long ago. But, at the same time, as a former teacher, she must be aware that she is both teaching and writing history with her literally hundreds of columns for the *Greenfield Recorder*.

So as Ruby Hemenway noodles possible subjects for another column and as Bob Gunn banks his plane to line up for that first spraying pass of the day, Barbara Coburn may be checking out her aqualung preparatory to entering the water carrying a shiny new brass propeller. And when she sees, through her goggles under water, the old "prop," wounded from its encounter with a hidden rock, she feels that satisfaction that comes from knowing that she can make the

---

*Reprinted with permission, *The Greenfield Recorder*.

vessel seaworthy again. Enough satisfaction for a day? In truth, more than all too many of any age will derive from today.

At the beginning of this chapter, I asked you to be critical of your own life. Of course, I mean like a drama critic, music critic, or a literary critic when they assess a piece of work as great, mediocre, or deplorable. If your life gets a rave review, if you find yourself like the fortunate people we have been reading about, I offer you my heartiest congratulations. Keep it up; keep living; and keep enjoying! If, however, you give yourself something less than a rave review, I suggest you contemplate the concept of change. For a couple of decades now, the thinkers have been stating with some pride that we live in an age of change! When did we not, I would be interested to know? But as universal as change has been, human beings have as universally tended to resist it. "Objects at rest tend to remain at rest." Yet there are plenty of exceptions. My own physician, in his late forties, has just quit medicine to enter law school. Police officers have become authors, firefighters have become artists, business executives have become farmers. Maybe the "thinkers" are right, change is rampant in the air here in the eighties and all comers are welcome. The other part of Newton's law states, "Objects in motion tend to remain in motion." That is highly descriptive of the people we've met in these pages. Perhaps the problem is, for those of us whose lives rate something less than a rave review, to "beam ourselves up" from the state of "at rest" to the state of "in motion." This may be the hardest part of improving the quality of your life but at least take heart from the fact that once "in motion" you'll tend to continue that way.

What kind of motion? There is only one person alive on this planet today who can answer that question. But answer it you must if you are determined to raise the quality of your life in line with the people you've been reading about. This is not to say that you must start painting or wood carving or lobbying in Washington or teaching English as a second language. To make a choice like that, I believe, would be putting the cart before the horse. The first step will be to make a determination of what quality, among those we looked at in each chapter, may be most lacking from your life. Examine your own

Enjoy

life as it has unfolded for the past year or two with regard to that particular quality.

For a trial run, let's take "variety." Think about the events of the past twenty-four months in terms of the variety of people you've been in contact with, the variety of places you have visited or lived in, the variety of activities you have engaged in. This is, of course, an analytical process. You may find that you're doing fine in the variety department. But let's suppose you're not. Let's suppose that your VQ (right—variety quotient) seems to be on the low side. Now, you switch from the analytical to the creative process.

To create, your mind needs stimulation; and stimulation is exactly the purpose for which the chapter on variety was written. At this point, I recommend you read "Variety" again with, perhaps, a little more care than the first time. Listen carefully to what each of the people says. Take Viola Dolzani, "That's really like medicine—yes, that's like medicine." Remember what she was talking about? Right. "When you're traveling, you forget about all your problems. And you meet so many nice people, you know." Maybe there's nothing you dislike more than travel. Travel has no monopoly on being able to provide variety. Listen carefully to what the other people in the chapter have to say to you—always trying to relate their life experiences to your life potential.

Thinking, dreaming, planning, supposing, are all pleasant ways of avoiding action. But enter Sir Isaac Newton into your life. The time has come to proceed from "at rest" to "in motion." If you've decided to try travel as the way to add variety to your life; if you've decided to visit that daughter in Houston; if you've decided to take the cruise to Alaska; if you've decided to go to Atlantic City or Lake Tahoe for two days, the magic moment arrives when you actually write a check for the down payment on your ticket. YOU ARE NOW IN MOTION!

Frightening, isn't it? That's how it strikes me. Frightening but also exciting. Exhilarating is a better word. Your life has now taken on a new dimension. Something new is beginning.

And life is what is beginning. Always beginning. Every morning after you've taken the step, you'll awaken to a true beginning. Because

LIFE BEGINS AT SIXTY

that is what living really is—beginning. Always the first step of a new journey, the first hour of a new day, the first words spoken in a new relationship, the first brush stroke on a new canvas. These things that mark beginnings, these are the things that take courage, these are the things that living is made of.

THE BEGINNING

Appendix

Some Organizations Whose Purpose Is to Assist Older Americans and Canadians

American Association of Homes for the Aging
1050 17th Street NW
Suite 770
Washington, DC 20036

Telephone: (202) 296-5960

Publishes *Nonprofit Provider News*, monthly. Provides information on housing for the elderly.

American Association of Retired Persons
1909 K Street NW
Washington, DC 20049

Telephone: (202) 872-4700

Western offices:
215 Long Beach Boulevard
Long Beach, CA 90801

Telephone: (213) 432-5781

Publishes *Modern Maturity,* bi-monthly, and "AARP News Bulletin," monthly. Provides a wide range of information and services for senior citizens.

Grandparents Anonymous
1924 Beverly
Sylvan Lake, MI 48053

Telephone: (313) 682-8384

Provides information on maintaining welfare of grandchildren and legal visitation rights of grandparents. Researches visitation rights in all states.

Gray Panthers
3635 Chestnut Street
Philadelphia, PA 10104

Telephone: (215) 382-3300

Publishes *The Network Newspaper,* bi-monthly. Aims to combat agism and discrimination against the old.

Jewish Association for Services for the Aged
40 West 68th Street
New York, NY 10023

Telephone: (212) 724-3200

Provides services necessary for the elderly to remain in their own communities. (New York and environs.)

Legal Counsel for the Elderly
1909 K Street NW
Washington, DC 20049

Telephone: (202) 728-4333

Provides free legal assistance to Washington residents sixty and over. (Affiliated with AARP.)

National Association of Senior Citizens
2525 Wilson Boulevard
Arlington, VA 22201

Telephone: (703) 241-1533

Publishes *Senior Guardian,* monthly, and *Our Age,* bi-monthly. Offers a wide range of services for seniors.

National Association of Area Agencies on Aging
600 Maryland Avenue SW
Washington, DC 20024

Telephone: (202) 484-7520

Publishes "The Point of Delivery," monthly newsletter. Members are Area Agencies on Aging established under provisions of the "Older Americans Act of 1965."

National Caucus and Center on Black Aged
1424 K Street NW, Suite 500
Washington, DC 20005

Telephone: (202) 637-8400

Publishes "Golden Age" newsletter, quarterly. Forty-five local groups in the United States; seeks to enhance the quality of life for blacks.

National Council on the Aging
600 Maryland Avenue SW
Washington, DC 20024

Telephone: (202) 479-1200

Publishes *Senior Center Report*, monthly. Broad membership of professionals offering information and other services to both organizations and individuals.

National Council of Senior Citizens
925 15th Street NW
Washington, DC 20005

Telephone: (202) 347-8800

Publishes *Senior Citizens News,* monthly. Organization of 4,000 senior citizen clubs, associations, etc.

National Institute on Aging
Building 31, Room 5C 35
9000 Rockville Pike
Bethesda, MD 20892

Telephone: (301) 496-1752

Federal research organization publishing a wide variety of health education material for older adults.

National Senior Citizens Law Center
1424 16th Street NW
Washington, DC 20036

Telephone: (202) 232-6570

Publishes a weekly newsletter. Is a legal services support center specializing in legal problems of the elderly.